The Mindful Diabetic:

Transform Your Type 2 Diabetes through Mindfulness

By Nikki Buamah

the use of any form of medication without the advice of their doctor or practitioner, but the book gives general information that could help in the wellbeing of the individual.

For more information, email nikki@nikkibuamahcoaching.com.

Get Your Free Gift

8 Simple Tips on Becoming More Mindful

To get the best experience with this book, I've found readers who download and use "8 simple tips on becoming more mindful" can implement faster and take the next steps needed to become a better version of themselves.

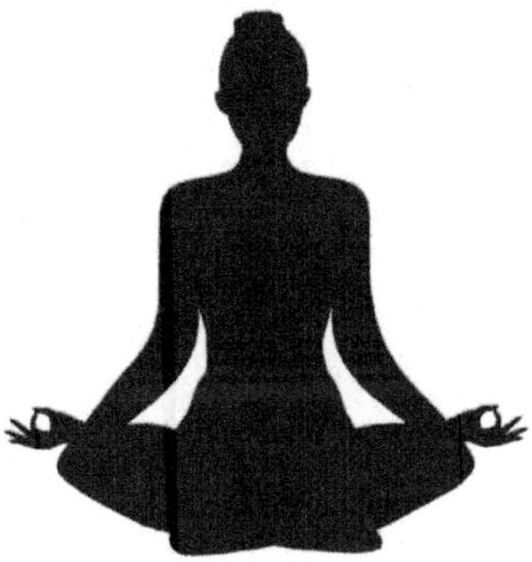

You can get a copy by visiting:

nikkibuamahcoaching.com

Dedication

To the dearest gifts of my life:

my children, Tamara and Michael

And

my husband, Francis

for their love, encouragement, and support

Foreword

I've known Nikki for more than 25 years, which is almost as long as I have been involved in looking after people with diabetes. It is, therefore, a great honour for me to have been asked to write the foreword to this book. In my job as a consultant in diabetes, I am aware of all of the pharmacological and technological advances that have been made over that time which have helped to reduce the devastating impact that the condition has on the people living with diabetes and their families. In that time, a myriad of new drugs have appeared on the market that have undergone rigorous clinical trials, showing that they help reduce the risk of premature cardiovascular death in people with diabetes. The advent of devices to continuously measure glucose concentrations or to deliver a constant infusion of insulin, devices that "talk" to each other to improve glucose control and to help minimise the impact of high or low blood glucose concentrations have helped people all over the world. These changes are to be celebrated by the health care professionals looking after the people with diabetes, as well as those living with the condition.

One of the things that the newer drugs and technology have done is to help reduce the worry and anxiety that people with diabetes live with daily. However, despite all of these advances, there remains a lot of work to do. The psychological effects on people having a long-term condition like diabetes are well recognised, yet there are very few institutions that can offer the appropriate level of mental health support they need or for all the people who need it. In the past, when there have been gaps in the ability of health care providers to deliver the care needed, it has fallen on the individuals themselves to come up with solutions; an example is the development of "open" artificial pancreas systems where people with diabetes themselves developed the software to allow them to manipulate the devices available to deliver better care and made them it freely available to anyone. Addressing the psychological needs of people living with diabetes is another area of need.

Many people living with diabetes know how stressful having the condition is and how that stress can adversely affect their glucose control. Anything that helps an individual to overcome the day-to-day struggles and, minimise or reduce the stresses that having a long-term condition brings can only be good. The mindfulness approach that Nikki advocates to self-managing diabetes advocated in this book is to be welcomed. I commend this book to you, and trust that you enjoy reading it as much as I did.

Professor Ketan Dhatariya MBBS MSc MD MS FRCP PhD

Consultant in Diabetes, Endocrinology and General Medicine

Norfolk and Norwich University Hospitals NHS Foundation Trust. Norwich Medical School

Table of Contents

Introduction

"Circumstances determined your past. The present is embracing you, and only you can define your future." —Terisita Marsal-Avila.

It's so commonly talked about, overweight and obesity is a pandemic, ever expanding, to the ends of the earth. It's gradually creeping into many households, a silent killer that, many times, goes unnoticed until it's too late. It's the major cause of type 2 diabetes in our modern world.

Nedu is a stockbroker, he leaves home for work quite early in the morning and finishes late in the evening. He's father to Sasha who is 4 years old. He gets back just in time to read her a bedtime story. Sasha eagerly awaits his return. Anytime he's late getting home, which is frequent, he would come back with guilty treats in the form of sweets or chocolates to pacify her. Nedu always felt guilty for not spending more time with his daughter. Sasha nibbles on her sweets as she tells her daddy all about her day at school, before he settles her down to sleep with his story telling or reading to her one of her favourite books. It was the same routine most days, and at weekends there were friends' parties with so much to eat, or family take aways of pizza, burgers, curries, you name it. As mum finds herself very busy during the week, she's quite happy to put her feet up at the weekends. Rich food was always the heart of celebration in Sasha's household. It wasn't a surprise that these habits continued into adulthood and Sasha acquired the nickname, 'Candy'. I'll let you guess the rest of Sasha's story as she turned forty-one.

In my professional practice as a clinical pharmacist and an advanced clinical practitioner working in general practice, I have a special interest in diabetes. I have seen lots of individuals who have been overwhelmed by the diagnosis of diabetes. Some remain in denial for a very long time while some others fight a losing battle with diabetes control. I've studied many patients, their patterns, and their lifestyles, read a lot of books, listened to podcasts, talked to affected friends and family, and researched a lot on diabetes care. I've come up with some answers, but despite this, some questions remain unanswered.

What's the reason for our increasing girth? Why do we eat the way we eat? We find out that a lot is triggered from childhood by our family, both immediate and extended, friends we've grown up with, school mates, the environment, social media, and our individual choices and decisions.

This book introduces how our mindset and mindful practice in various aspects of our lives can change both our internal and external behaviours, affecting how we think and everything we do. It shows how creating new habits can positively have an impact on our blood glucose levels. I only started practicing meditation and mindfulness a few years ago but I know for a certainty that the experience of calm and being present in the moment will enable people living with diabetes to control their lives better. You'll also come to this conviction as you read along.

As a child, my mother encouraged fasting at certain times of the year on religious grounds. This ritual was open to translation with no food or drink before 12 noon or longer if you could. I kind of dreaded these seasons. It was seen as a religious act, but I interpreted it as starvation. The human mind is funny, as, sometimes, one can go without eating for long periods if it's not forced upon you. But once it's formalised, that's when the craving kicks in. Fast-forward to adulthood, I now see it as a great way to reset my system to its baseline, giving the body time to be in its natural state without constantly forcing it into the action of breaking down and digesting everything I throw at it. I call this intermittent fasting.

There have been so many publications on diabetes in relation to weight loss and exercise. A lot of findings have been published in diabetes journals and websites such as the Diabetes UK, NHS website, American Diabetic Association, European Journals, *BMJ*, *JAMA*, and there have been open discussions on diabetes. The hope is that the information out there will help make people's lives better. It's unclear what percentage of this information is seen or read by the public and taken on to make a difference. I would say 90% is pretty much ignored but the struggle continues for diabetes awareness and education. This book has brought together through a summary of practices that are proven to work if you put in the time and dedication. Actions must be repeated before habits are formed. I hope they'll work for you. They're simple to adopt anywhere, anytime, and I encourage you to read it right to the end. You'll gain the results you desire and form lasting good habits to serve you in other aspects of your life.

This is not a diet book. There's nothing here about counting calories or specific recipes. It's more about finding the right mindset and mindfulness practice to feel empowered and confident in your ability to take control of your health, to help in the quest to reverse your diabetes or get it under tight control, to live a fulfilling live and avoid the complications associated with uncontrolled diabetes. This book won't give you six pack abs or make you a catwalk model; however, it will move you in the right direction towards health and wellness. I've focused on adults with type 2 diabetes who are between 40 and 55 years, as research indicates that more people are diagnosed around this age bracket, although anyone can read this book and find at least one area that will be of benefit to them. It's an easy-to-read guide. It will give you focus and calmness and help you get centred. If you've picked this book up and have been a type 2 diabetic for 6 years or less, then this is the book for you. It's easier to control diabetes in the earlier stages. Be sure to read it. If your diabetes is advanced in years, you'll still benefit from aspects of the book, since we can all benefit from a shift of our mindset and become mindful at any stage in our lives. We must believe this is possible and that we can create a better story for ourselves where it becomes part and parcel of our daily living, and you'll see how it impacts you and everyone around you.

My initial thought before I started writing this book was to start a weekly or daily blog about my thoughts. I feel compiling it into a book as a one stop for all is a great idea too. There are four parts to this book. It's not written in a linear way, so you can choose any part to read first.

Part 1: I write about the meaning of diabetes and why we develop diabetes. The important role of insulin and how it regulates what we eat.

Part 2: Why having the right mindset is the ultimate way to achieve the results you desire and how this can be developed.

Part 3: Mindfulness, the act of being present in the now moment. How being mindful can reduce stress, anxiety, and depression, and ultimately reduce blood glucose levels. I also write about how sleep is an important factor in regulating blood glucose control, as too little sleep can increase insulin resistance.

Part 4: Other mindful practices that can play a significant role in managing and controlling blood sugar levels which ultimately will make you a better individual overall.

Finally, it's time to make a move on your health and wellbeing. It's never too late, and it's possible if you act. Are you a diabetic or have a friend or family member with diabetes, or are you just curious for the sake of knowledge? You'll find as you page through this book, your brain will be triggered to seek out more practical steps for application. Some of the examples I've given in this book might be you. We're all different and it takes different triggers to get us going. Use this to positively impact your wellbeing. I wish you well in your quest for health and knowledge.

Chapter 1: Diabetes

Scaling figures

According to the World Population Review, as of 2021, approximately 10% of all people aged 20-79 in the world, or 537 million people, were living with diabetes. The website predicts that this number will increase to 643 million by 2030 and to 783 million by 2045. The World Health Organization (WHO, 2012) also stated that diabetes was directly responsible for the deaths of 1.5 million people in the same year. The International Diabetic Federation (IDF) also stated that in the IDF Africa Region, diabetes is the cause of 416,000 deaths in 2021, while hyperglycaemia in pregnancy affects 1 in 8 live births

Diabetes can lead to a number of complications, such as heart attacks, strokes, kidney failure, blindness, and leg amputations. The Centres for Disease Control and Prevention (CDC) suggest that 1 in 3 Americans have prediabetes, and over 80% are unaware that they have it.

Diabetes simply unravelled

"Insulin is not a cure for diabetes; it is a treatment. It enables the diabetic to burn sufficient carbohydrates so that proteins and fats may be added to the diet in sufficient quantities to provide energy for the economic burdens of life." —Frederick Banting

Diabetes is a condition where there's continuously high levels of sugar (glucose) in the blood. A lot of foods we eat contain sugar and carbohydrates, which the body will use for energy. The body needs sugar as the fuel to perform and complete mundane things in life like walking, breathing, dancing. With diabetes, it's difficult to control glucose, which needs to be carried from the blood stream to the cells for energy. We need a special hormone called insulin. Insulin is a peptide hormone that plays a key part in blood glucose regulation of carbohydrates, protein, and fat. It's vital for the transfer process of glucose to the cells. Insulin acts as a key to unlock the doors for glucose to enter into the cells. Insulin is released from the pancreas. The pancreas is an organ that houses the beta cells that release insulin.

In type 2 diabetes, the body builds up resistance to insulin and more insulin is needed to bring down blood glucose levels. As a result, the pancreas needs to produce more insulin than it would normally need to. If the pancreas can no longer produce enough insulin to bring down sugar levels, symptoms of diabetes will begin to develop.

Type 2 diabetes comes on gradually and it can take years for symptoms to appear. Further development of type 2 diabetes can lead to loss of insulin producing beta cells from the pancreas, they 'burn out', which can lead to the need for insulin to be administered. When the pancreas is out of action, blood glucose levels rise uncontrollably. The longer we've had diabetes, the more difficult it is for us to go into remission.

Let us look at this in a different context, as diabetes is a complex condition and can be described in different ways. A condition in which the body's ability to produce or even respond to the hormone insulin is weakened or damaged, causing abnormal metabolism of carbohydrates and elevated levels of glucose in the blood. When the body can no longer produce enough or any insulin, it's called type 1 diabetes, and it's not related to age or weight. Such individuals will need immediate glucose control with insulin.

Imagine you have 100 lockers in a room with a pile of keys in a bowl and you must identify which key fits to open each locker. Assuming this process is automated, a key is fed in but bounces out because it's the wrong fit. Sometimes, the right key fits, it opens and allows entry of glucose into the cells. As a result of this trial and error, not enough glucose is going in, leading to excess glucose left in the blood stream. Insulin is the keys. You might have enough insulin (keys), but the body cells don't respond as they should. When the insulin that's produced isn't enough or doesn't work effectively, just like having the wrong keys to open the gate for glucose entry into the cells, we call this type 2 diabetes. The American Diabetic Association has defined hyperglycaemia or high blood sugar as inadequate glucose transfer into the cells, causing excessive residual glucose in the bloodstream.

Insulin resistance (IR) is a condition where the body stops responding to insulin. The excess glucose in the blood then reduces the ability of the cells to absorb and use blood sugar for energy. This driving factor leads to increased risk of developing prediabetes, and eventually, type 2 diabetes. Insulin resistance is mostly associated with tiredness, cravings, and weight gain; however, one can be insulin resistant without being overweight. Insulin resistance can be reversed through lifestyle changes.

There are other types of diabetes. I mentioned Type 1 diabetes earlier, which commonly occurs at a younger age and less commonly at an older age. Some scientists call it juvenile or, more appropriately, autoimmune diabetes. Gestational diabetes occurs in pregnancy and would usually resolve once the child is born. However, regular monitoring is required as such individuals have a high risk of developing type 2 diabetes in the future. Type 3c diabetes is called pancreatogenesis diabetes, as this form of diabetes occurs secondary to pancreatic disease. I'll be focusing on type 2 diabetes in this book.

Double trouble

Have you heard of the word 'diabesity'? It has been defined in the Oxford dictionary as a form of diabetes that typically develops in later life and is associated with being obese. However, a modification of this definition is required, as people are developing diabesity at a much younger age due to our unhealthy lifestyle choices. Living a sedentary life with minimal physical activity is one of the contributory factors to obesity. Being overweight is certainly a risk factor for type 2 diabetes.

Our diet, fast foods, convenient take aways, prepacked ready meals, frozen or unfrozen, contain very high sugar (glucose, fructose) and salt content. An article from the *Journal of Nutrition* (as cited in Harvard T.H. Chan School of Public Health, n.d.) reported that consumption of refined carbohydrates with a high glycaemic index, such as white bread or white rice, increases the risk of type 2 diabetes. Conversely, consuming whole grains, such as bran cereal and oatmeal, can reduce the risk. Refined carbohydrates are foods that have had the outer layers, such as bran and germ, removed from the grain, leaving only the starchy endosperm. Other examples of refined carbohydrates are pastries, sweets and candy, sugary drinks, breakfast cereals, and processed snacks. Refined carbohydrates can cause a rapid spike in blood sugar levels, and consuming them in excess can lead to weight gain, which can lead to type 2 diabetes and other health problems like high cholesterol. It's important to limit refined carbohydrates and choose whole grains instead, which are more nutritious and can help to regulate blood sugar levels.

When we drink alcohol in large amounts, the cells sensitivity to insulin decreases. Excessive alcohol consumption can also cause pancreatitis, which is a common side effect of diabetes. Drinking without limits results in a high chance of increasing body weight and progressing obesity. Alcoholism is high on the list of an unhealthy lifestyle choice. Its high sugar and calorie content combined with reduced activity can damage the liver, which helps in regulating blood sugar. Alcohol acts as an aperitif (appetizer) to stimulate appetite before a meal, and diabetics may find that they crave food quite frequently with increased alcohol consumption. There's the common belief that consumption of beer in large amounts determines an individual's waist circumference. A few studies conducted on alcohol intake, when reviewed, had varying results on its relationship with weight gain. Smith et al. (2018) suggested that there is an overall weight gain, which is not specific to the abdomen. Lee et al. (2019) also suggested that drinking beer at more than 500ml daily, even though the strength was not specified, might be associated with abdominal obesity, while recent research by Shen et al. (2021) states that there is evidence to suggest that abdominal obesity may increase the risk of hip fractures. Just to put this in context and in a lighter mood, beer belly isn't just from drinking beer, it stems mostly from what we eat and our activity levels. And the terminologies can expand to phrases like middle-age spread, spare tire, or even apple shape. Abdominal obesity is a health risk that can lead to diabetes, heart disease, and erectile dysfunction.

Tobacco smoking can increase your risk of type 2 diabetes by 30–40% or can worsen it if you already have this condition. We read how insulin helps the blood sugar get into the cells. Nicotine from smoking modifies cells so they cease to respond to insulin; this, in turn, increases the blood sugar levels. Toxic chemicals in cigarettes can harm the cells in the body and cause inflammation, stopping the cells from responding to insulin and leading to development of cancerous cells. Smokers tend to have increased belly fat even though they can have lower body mass than nonsmokers.

About 40-80% of people with diabetes have hypertension or are twice likely to develop hypertension with diabetes. This is important to note as hypertension quite often goes unnoticed and can present without symptoms. I would encourage everyone to have a blood pressure monitor at home and know your numbers. Values of less than 140mmHg systolic and less than 80mmHg diastolic pressure are recommended. The combination of diabetes and hypertension can significantly increase the risks of kidney disease, heart disease, heart attack, stroke, retinopathy, and lack of blood circulation to the peripheral areas of the body, causing foot and nerve damage.

Cholesterol (lipids) is important for overall health, but hyperlipidaemia, meaning high cholesterol levels manifests when the bad cholesterol, low density lipoprotein, and triglyceride levels become too high. As diabetes can damage the lining of the arteries, cholesterol very quickly sticks on, leading to a build-up of fatty deposits that cause the arteries to narrow or get blocked. Studies have shown that there's a link between low levels of good cholesterol, high density lipoprotein, and glucose intolerance or abnormal glucose (Katz, 2018; NCD Risk Factor Collaboration, 2016). If the good cholesterol is increased, diabetic risk may be reduced. Foods containing olive oil, whole grains, beans, high-fibre foods like fruits and vegetables are great examples of foods that lower bad cholesterol, which will inversely increase high density lipoprotein, the good cholesterol.

Other risks of type 2 diabetes include family history (genes), history of gestational diabetes, and polycystic ovary syndrome (PCOS). Seventy-five percent of children with type 2 diabetes have a close relative who has it, either due to genetics, or shared lifestyle habits. Having a parent or sibling with type 2 diabetes is linked with an increased risk.

Recognising the signs

Diabetes is usually picked up through screening (blood glucose or HBA1c test) which had been recommended by a doctor or clinician during an investigation for a complication, when annual health checks are done, or for diabetic signs and symptoms presented by the person. Diabetes screening tells you if you have diabetes or how serious it is. If your family member has diabetes or you're at risk of developing diabetes, it's good practice to start screening early even in the absence of any symptoms. In the United Kingdom (UK), the National Health Service

(NHS) provides health checks that screen for type 2 diabetes and assess an individual's risk of developing the condition. These checks are recommended for people aged forty and above. Do contact your doctor or healthcare professional immediately for a medical check-up if you are already this age or are experiencing any of the symptoms detailed below.

Thirst - Getting thirsty all the time occurs as the kidney tries to filter out the excess glucose, leading to frequent urination especially at night.

Tiredness and hunger, particularly after meals, occurs due to the inability of the glucose in the blood to be absorbed into the cells for energy.

The vision gets blurry as the tiny blood vessels in the eyes get damaged due to hyperglycaemia.

Wounds and cuts become slow to heal due to damaged nerves and lack of adequate blood flow. Includes itchiness of the skin, especially around the genitals.

There might be sudden weight loss or muscle mass loss.

Certain skin disorders, such as psoriasis or acanthosis nigricans (dark velvety patches in skin folds and creases), can occur.

Be aware of the less common symptoms of nausea and dizziness that could also be a sign of diabetes.

Prediabetes is when glucose levels are raised but not to the point of becoming diabetic. The centres for disease control and prevention recon that about 96 million adults in America, which is 1 in 3 adults have prediabetes and greater than 80% are unaware they have it. Prediabetes should be a wakeup call to act. Don't Delay! Talk to a Clinician! Get Tested! Act!

Diagnosis of diabetes

Candy, 41 years old with a family history of diabetes, attended a routine health check screening. Both her mum and aunty were diabetic. She weighed 89kg. Candy booked to see a clinician as she was getting regular headaches which were worse at night, and she was waking up three or four times at night to pass urine. She had been taking paracetamol which helped with her headaches but only for a short while. Candy's headache was always in the background until she took her next dose of pain killers. She got fed-up with the headaches and disturbed sleep and decided to see her doctor. Her blood pressure when checked was high. Her blood glucose level was also significantly raised at 20mmol/l when checked. Her doctor referred her to have some blood tests done. Candy's results came back, confirming a diagnosis of type 2 diabetes. It was only then that she recognised that her other played-down symptoms of continued dry mouth and blurry vision were all connected to diabetes. Her diabetic journey began.

Type 2 diabetes is a lifelong condition that can be reversed or tightly controlled. It develops gradually over the years as it creeps into your life unnoticed. Then, suddenly, it becomes more serious. Type 2 diabetes is commonly diagnosed during routine examinations or tests for unrelated conditions as previously mentioned. High cholesterol and being overweight is an indication that you might be heading in that direction. Thousands of people are carrying diabetic loads without realising it. It's vital not to assume that minor deterioration in health is because of a natural ageing process.

Diagnosis of type 2 diabetes might come as a shock even though you may have someone in the family who has diabetes. Somehow, we feel it won't happen to us. Some people might feel scared, angry, alone, or even ashamed of the diagnosis. Some may need time to digest and could go through stages similar to the grieving process of shock and denial, anger, bargaining, guilt, depression, reconstruction, then acceptance. How long it takes to accept will depend on the individual, the support groups they have around them, the healthcare professional's input, and their willingness to accept or access help. Various support groups can remove the feeling of being alone. You can join diabetic forums like Diabetes UK, the American Diabetic Association (ADA), or many other national and local forums or organisations around the world. Your doctor or healthcare specialist can refer you to structured diabetes educational classes and psychological care that you might need to develop confidence, courage, and resilience, thus enabling you to take positive steps towards reversing or controlling diabetes.

Getting Tested: Diagnosis takes place when there are two instances of elevated blood glucose levels, indicated by HbA1C readings of 48mmol/l (6.5%) or higher, or blood glucose level readings of 7.7mmol/l or higher, obtained through blood testing. The HbA1C testing measures the amount of glucose that attaches to a specific type of haemoglobin called A1C. Haemoglobin A1C (HbA1C) is a type of haemoglobin, which is a protein found in red blood cells (RBCs) that carries oxygen throughout the body. When glucose (sugar) enters the bloodstream, it binds to haemoglobin molecules in RBCs. HbA1C is a form of haemoglobin that has glucose attached to it, and the amount of HbA1C in the blood reflects the average blood glucose level over the past 2-3 months. Or, to put differently, HbA1C test measures the percentage of haemoglobin that is bound to glucose in the blood. This test is often used to monitor blood sugar control in diabetes. Because RBCs have a lifespan of about 120 days, the HbA1C test provides an average of blood glucose levels over this time period, rather than just a snapshot of blood glucose at the time of the test. It forms a stable bond known as a glycated A1C molecule (Smith, 2021). The lower the result, the better the control of blood sugar and the lower the risk of complications. HbA1c is the diagnostic test used in a lot of countries. Fewer countries use the fasting blood glucose test. If you're anaemic, relying on HbA1c alone can lead to a false or inappropriate diagnosis. A full blood count (FBC) would go hand in hand with the A1c test, and if anaemic, the cause and treatment should be addressed. The FBC test typically measures several different components of the blood, like the red blood cells, and by analysing the results of an FBC test, healthcare providers can gain important information about a person's health and act on these results.

Early detection of diabetes cannot be overemphasised. Much more awareness is needed about early detection. If you're aged 40 years and over, in United Kingdom, you're eligible for a free NHS health check. Earlier checks can be done if you pick up early signs. In females who have had gestational diabetes, yearly checks are encouraged as they're at a higher risk of developing diabetes. If you have a family history of diabetes, you'll be encouraged to have an earlier check.

Story: Forty-year-old Jack, was a busy professional. He had always been in good health and didn't think much about his diet or exercise routine. One day, when he went to see his doctor for a routine check-up, he was told that his blood sugar levels were high and that he had been diagnosed with type 2 diabetes.

Jack was shocked and confused, he had no idea how this could have happened to him. He had never had any symptoms and had never thought about the fact that he might be at risk for diabetes.

His doctor explained to him that type 2 diabetes often develops gradually and without symptoms, which is why it's often referred to as a "silent killer." He also explained that type 2 diabetes is often linked to lifestyle factors such as being overweight or obese, having a family history of diabetes, and being physically inactive.

Jack realized that his busy lifestyle and poor diet had caught up with him. He knew that he needed to make some changes to manage his diabetes and improve his health. He attended the diabetic education class and with the help of his doctor, Jack made some changes to his lifestyle. He started to exercise regularly, eat a healthy diet, and monitor his blood sugar levels. He also made a point to respond to regular calls for check-ups.

Jack's story shows that type 2 diabetes can develop gradually and without symptoms, and it's important to be aware of the risk factors and to make lifestyle changes to prevent or manage the condition. With the right support and guidance, it's possible to improve health and manage diabetes effectively.

Chapter 2: The Mindset Game - How Our Thoughts Affect Us

"Action is a great restorer and builder of confidence. Inaction is not only the result, but the cause, of fear. Perhaps the action you take will be successful; perhaps different action or adjustments will have to follow. But any action is better than no action at all." —Norman Vincent Peale

Mindset! Is this a BUZZWORD? There's so much talk about having the right mindset. The various definitions of mindset all point to beliefs, attitudes, thoughts, emotions, needs, and how they affect your behaviour, actions, or outcomes. I was interested in finding out how different dictionaries described these words that we so frequently use interchangeably. According to Tony Robins, a belief is a feeling of certainty about something. For example, if I believe I can reverse my diabetes, what I'm saying is, "I feel certain that I can reverse my diabetes." B.F. Skinner describes thoughts as behaviours we haven't learned to observe yet. According to the *Oxford Dictionary*, an attitude is a settled way of thinking or feeling about someone or something, typically one that's reflected in a person's behaviour. The *Cambridge Dictionary* defines mindset as a person's way of thinking or their opinions. The free dictionary has a slightly different definition, describing mindset as a fixed mental attitude or disposition that predetermines a person's responses to interpretations or situations. An inclination or a habit. The *World English Dictionary* defines mindset as "the ideas and attitudes with which a person approaches a situation, especially when these are seen as being difficult to alter."

Wikipedia gives its own Mindset description as *"a set of assumptions, methods, or notations held by one or more people or groups of people that is so established that it creates a powerful incentive within these people or groups to continue to adopt or accept prior behaviours, choices, or tools."*

Which definition resonates more with you?

Mindset is formed through experiences, things that have happened, things that were taught to us. These could be cultural, or community based, positive or negative, and combined with your personal interpretation of those experiences.

In her book New Psychology of Success, Carol Dweck, a professor of psychology, discusses the concept of fixed and growth mindsets. A fixed mindset is characterized by the belief that an individual's abilities are set in stone and their basic qualities, such as intelligence or talent, are fixed traits. They're stuck in childhood experiences and old paradigms, spending a lot of time recording their intelligence or talent instead of growing them. They believe that talent alone will create success without effort of improvement.

Someone with a growth mindset believes that growth and development are possible and has a willingness to take on new challenges. They understand that mistakes or failures can happen but are still motivated to continually look for and try new learning or strategy.

The person with a fixed mindset will accept that diabetes is genetic or runs in the family and will decide not to act and take control when diagnosed with diabetes. It can be viewed as a burden This person gives up easily, feels helpless and hopeless, finding every excuse not to address the issue. Instead, they accept medication in the initial stages without a conscious effort to try to manage/reverse diabetes naturally. Some are reluctant to seek advice from healthcare professionals, aren't keen to learn but crave sympathy of others to accept and understand that diabetes is here, and nothing can be done about it, and remain in a victim mode. A person with a fixed mindset won't engage with healthcare professionals to work towards a goal, thinking, *Why should I bother*! You might remember the story of the elephant mindset. The full-grown elephants still believed that they could not break away from the same ropes that were tied to their feet when they were young and small, strong enough to keep them in place at that young age. Another great story, using the hare and the tortoise as an example, is that a person with a fixed mindset may believe that the hare's natural speed and talent make him inherently better than the tortoise, and, therefore, he will always win. On the other hand, a person with a growth mindset may see the tortoise's perseverance and determination as something that can be learned and improved upon, allowing him to eventually surpass the hare. In other words, a person with a fixed mindset may believe that their abilities are predetermined and unchangeable, while a person with a growth mindset believes that their abilities can be developed through effort and hard work.

Your mindset will influence and ultimately determine what you do and don't do, how you act, and how you react.

From experience, some people find acceptance, and readiness to address diabetes takes a long time, but I have found that developing the right mindset always tips the scale in the positive direction. If you view yourself negatively, your outcomes will be worse. Positive outcomes can be achieved through a growth mindset. Consistently and persistently making an effort to maintain healthy blood sugar levels can reduce the risk of complications and improve overall quality of life. This can lead to a sense of empowerment and control, as you take an active role in your own health and well-being.

Let's talk medication

This, however, may not be the solution. Taking medication can sometimes make us lazy. Accepting pills without addressing the root cause can, in the interim, keep your diabetes under control, but your condition will slowly and progressively get worse. More or different medicines will be added on to maintain such control. Hence one of the reasons diabetes is called the silent killer, as diabetes is progressive. Just to clarify, the term "silent killer" is used before diagnosis when we're not aware that we have diabetes and living an unhealthy lifestyle without symptoms, also during therapy when we decide not to act and rely solely on medication to kick our condition. Medically, improvement of diabetes has always been viewed through a disease centred approach, through measurement of values such as glycated haemoglobin (HBA1c), blood pressure, cholesterol levels, and a few other parameters (Gæde et al., 2008). These are the gold standard in clinical practice. Relying on medication only without engaging in lifestyle changes for improvement can be a fixed mindset.

Heritability of excess sugars

Is Type 2 diabetes associated with heredity and heritability?

Can Type 2 diabetes can be inherited? What does this mean to you? Or is diabetes an interaction between environmental factors and a strong hereditary component? Is this a genuine excuse not to act? Environmental risk factors include obesity, sedentary lifestyle, small or large birth weight and stress. Toxins or other nutritional factors may also play a role. If one or both of your parents have or had diabetes doesn't mean that you'll develop diabetes. It does mean, however, that you have a greater chance of developing type 2 diabetes if you don't act. First-degree relatives of people with type 2 diabetes are at a higher risk compared with those without the condition in their family. A study published in *The World Journal of Diabetes* in 2013 described type 2 diabetes as the result of interaction between environmental factors and a strong hereditary component. There's still limited knowledge of heritability. With more research in the future, gene therapy and epigenetic reprogramming could prove a great way to alter the risk of diabetes. Epigenetics studies the changes that occurs in living organisms, in this case humans, which are caused by modification of gene expression instead of alteration of the genetic code itself. An awareness of family history can encourage steps to prevent type 2 diabetes and would help in an early diagnosis, which, in turn, will help in preventing complications that come with diabetes. With the knowledge of environmental factors, it's noted that everyone isn't impacted in the same way. With the same environmental exposures, some people are more susceptible to developing diabetes than others and this increased risk could be inherited. Lifestyle seems to be more influential than genes. Being aware of how genes and the environment, affect diabetes can encourage us to treat and manage the risk of complications.

Myths

A cross sectional study was carried out in a teaching hospital of Delhi, India in 2008 to get information on social demographics and myths about diabetes. The study involved diabetic patients, those who accompanied the patients, and others who were nondiabetics. Twenty-two percent said eating more sugar causes diabetes. Others said that diabetes can only occur in old age. Other more interesting myths were that soaking feet in water can help control blood sugar and diabetes is punishment for past sins and is cured by spiritual treatment. Of the diabetics interviewed, 12.1% were taking herbal medicines and some of these diabetics were unaware of the role diet and lifestyle play in controlling diabetes and that complications could occur if diabetes were uncontrolled. Even though this study was conducted over a decade ago, there still isn't enough awareness about type 2 diabetes.

Misconceptions

A recent study on diabetic patients in Taiwan which was published by the *Journal of Diabetes Research* in 2020 examined misconceptions of diabetes. The survey was in the form of a true or false questionnaire seeking to find out diabetic knowledge in different demographics in Taiwan. The most common misconception was that people always feel when their blood sugar level is high. Two others were that being a vegetarian helps control sugar levels and insulin administration hurts the kidneys, and, as a result, one might need dialysis. The total knowledge scores were associated with their education level, suggesting that individuals with higher levels of education had a better understanding of diabetes and its management compared to those with lower levels of education.

There's a big misconception that obesity and lack of exercise causes diabetes. Both can place you at a greater risk, but the main cause is insulin resistance, which can be a genetic factor. There are many obese individuals who don't have diabetes, and many who've never been obese end up being diabetic. A typical example is in the South Asian descent of India and China where there's a high rate of type 2 diabetes without obesity. Thin fat obesity phenotype is being metabolically unhealthy but not obese. It's said to happen when there's addition of fat to an already thin frame. The body mass index (BMI) when measured is normal but the percentage of body fat is high disproportionately based on ethnicity and gender. In the predecessors of these individuals during the rural-urban migration which might have caused people who were previously thin and super active physically to deposit fat due to a more sedentary lifestyle and could have been programmed genetically at foetal growth to produce offspring with such characteristics. This could just be one out of so many possible factors. The full genetics of type 2 diabetes is still unknown. Scientists have focused on the worsening function of the pancreas in many people to be the major cause of diabetes. New genetic variants keep increasing. So far about 32 novel genes have been identified that may increase diabetic risk. Identifying the genes related to the variants would be a breakthrough to better understand the physiology of diabetes and how to combat it. The thin fat obese person has a similar cardiometabolic risks as the obvious obese person. I have come across similar cases and have advised them to focus on the inside work of exercising and eating healthy, and not get complacent because the external looks good.

This misconception has led to a widespread belief that type 2 diabetes is a lifestyle disease, which, to some extent, it is in a lot of cases, but to generalise that lifestyle caused their condition is wrong. The misconception is common not only in the public perception but also in the healthcare system. In the UK, the government has a program for diabetes prevention when prediabetic diagnosis has been made, and the structured education class, when there's a definite type 2 diabetes diagnosis. These are based on lifestyle changes, as there's an assumption that being overweight and not getting enough exercise can cause type 2 diabetes, and that individuals can prevent the disease from progressing by modifying their lifestyle. Unfortunately, this assumption can cause individuals who already have type 2 diabetes to feel guilty and ashamed about their condition. One can argue that if 80% of people with type 2 diabetes developed their condition through lifestyle behaviour, then it makes sense to tackle these first. By targeting lifestyle factors such as diet and exercise, there is potential to prevent the development of type 2 diabetes as well as other chronic diseases such as high blood pressure, heart disease, and respiratory disease in a significant portion of the population. Additionally, addressing these factors may also improve the health outcomes of individuals who have already been diagnosed with the condition. However, it's important to consider that some cases of type 2 diabetes may have a genetic component or other underlying medical factors, and these cases may require different approaches to treatment and management. Nonetheless, addressing lifestyle factors should be a key aspect of any strategy to prevent and manage type 2 diabetes.

Chapter 3: The Widening Mindset

Healthy mindsets can influence how people perceive illness. A growth mindset could be linked to positive health outcomes. People with a fixed mindset of health will view illness more negatively and consequently have worse outcomes compared with those with a growth mindset who believe that health can be improved through effort. Our mindset determines the way we deal with tough situations. It's an improvement through practice even with great challenges.

A healthy mindset isn't just a positive mindset, it also means having a balanced healthy mindset when you're able to see the full picture, can make smart decisions and not be influenced by beliefs, role models you had as a child, people around you, and the environment that might be hurting you again. A growth mindset is inspired by success of others.

Mindset isn't predetermined. Anyone can choose a growth mindset and do the impossible. We can train our brain to learn with gradual repetitive steps.

Diagnosis of diabetes is certainly a life changer. Your growth mindset would want to make you improve.

Story: Forty-two-year-old Sarah attended for her yearly review. This time last year, she was struggling to manage her type 2 diabetes. She had a fixed mindset and believed that her condition was permanent and unchangeable. She felt helpless and didn't see the point in trying to make lifestyle changes.

When she met with me last year, I helped her understand the concept of a growth mindset. She learned that by adopting a growth mindset, she could view her diabetes as a challenge that could be managed through effort and learning.

With this new perspective, Sarah started making small changes to her lifestyle. She began to exercise regularly and made healthier food choices. She also started monitoring her blood sugar levels and communicating more with her healthcare team.

As a result, Sarah's diabetes began to improve. Her blood sugar levels became more stable, and she lost weight. She also found that she felt better overall. She realized that she had the power to manage her diabetes and improve her health. Sarah's story shows that a growth mindset can be a powerful tool for managing type 2 diabetes.

Acceptance commitment therapy (ACT)

While psychotherapy is not a treatment for diabetes itself, it can be a helpful tool for individuals with diabetes who may be struggling to cope with the demands of managing the condition. Diabetes can have a significant impact on an individual's mental health, and psychotherapy can provide them with a safe and supportive space to address any related emotional or psychological issues. For instance, therapy may help individuals with diabetes to better understand and manage their feelings of stress, anxiety, or depression related to their condition. Additionally, psychotherapy can help individuals with diabetes to identify and address any negative thought patterns or behaviours that may be hindering their ability to manage their condition effectively. Overall, incorporating psychotherapy into a comprehensive diabetes care plan may improve both physical and mental health outcomes for individuals living with this condition.

A new form of cognitive and behavioural therapy (CBT) called acceptance and commitment therapy has been explored in recent years which aims to increase "psychological flexibility" by using acceptance and mindfulness tactics together with a commitment and behavioural change approach. This I find interesting, as it covers most aspects of life and has led to positive health outcomes when applied in diabetic programmes. ACT makes people realise that it's normal to feel the way they feel psychologically, and they can learn and adopt a healthier lifestyle, which can make life richer just by changing their story and thoughts about diabetes. Through mindful action, we can create a meaningful life and overcome all sorts of barriers in the form of unpleasant experiences (thoughts, memories, sensations, feelings, visuals, etc.).

Psychological flexibility means that you can stay present with and, at the same time, adapt to challenges of life by taking useful action despite your thoughts or feelings and still stay true to your values or what's important to you. Let's look at this in 6 sections with examples of how this can be applied.

A. Knowing what to focus on and what to let go off. Learning as much as you can about diabetes, your type of diabetes. Becoming an expert on your condition.

B. Recognising when your behaviour isn't serving you and changing it. Am I eating the right foods, in the right proportion, at the right time?

C. Seeing when you might be wrong and changing a viewpoint such as the thought of not being able to lead a healthy normal life or not reversing diabetes through effort. Remember belief is a choice.

D. Finding the balance between different parts of your life. Replan your life to suit the new you. Empower yourself and change for yourself.

E. Continuing towards your goals even when you encounter setbacks. Failed exercise regimen? Pick yourself up and try the same again or something different.

F. Finding imaginative ways to deal with challenges whilst not compromising your values. How about baking and enjoying a sugar-free cake?

Inspirational tips

How do we take action?

I've drawn these inspirational tips from Jim Rohn, who was a well-known American entrepreneur, author, and motivational speaker. He famously said that motivation is what gets you started. It involves deciding, planning, starting, progressing, then achieving.

Decide - The day you decide to change a habit in any aspect of your life, eating, drinking, physical activity, sleeping, friendships, work, or business, could be a day you look back on over time as an important inspirational day in your life when the mind was ready to act. It's when you decided to choose a better diet for your health, longevity, and your family. Indecision will be putting off.

Plan - When you start a plan, so many thoughts come to you and ideas start taking shape. Best to put these on paper. Which of these can be done, as your life will have to change to some extent in adjusting to diabetes? These thoughts become real when put on paper. All these plans made will soon dwindle over time if action isn't taken.

Start - You would have planned before starting on this life-changing journey, deciding on your diet and whether you'll shop for the week and prep your meals ahead to free up time in the kitchen to eliminate the excuse of not enough time. You can opt to buy healthy frozen vegetables that can easily be warmed up. Say daily such as "I'm on a new track. I have carved out for myself a new beginning. I'll never be the same as before again. I'm leaving the old ways that didn't serve me behind and taking my first steps to better health." Start a new commitment to learning about diabetes. Surround yourself with information and inspiration; read books; go to reputable internet sites; watch videos; and join communities to listen, read, and learn from people's stories. Sign up for a class. Accept referrals to educational classes from your doctor or healthcare professional. If these opportunities aren't taken, you may lose motivation and not progress.

Progress - You have started. How are you progressing? There may be some excitement in progress. In terms of exercise, you might have started walking for just 10 minutes. Now you've increased to 20 or 30 minutes after a few weeks or you're jogging round the block and feel your breathing is better. Little at a time, you lose weight. You keep going and don't look back. You'll be happy with your progress. Unhappiness is the lack of progress towards a preset goal. Happiness is making progressive wins.

Achieve - You decided, you planned, you started, and you progressed. Now after setting your targets and following through, you're achieving. It might take weeks, months, years. You're in a better state of health, happier, and the future looks bright.

When you form a habit, it keeps you going. Jim Rohn's advice highlights the importance of motivation in initiating change but also emphasizes that lasting change requires the development of good habits. While motivation can inspire action, it may not be enough to sustain progress in the long term.

Know your numbers!

HbA1c is a marker that indicates your average blood sugar levels in the previous 3 months. It's also known as glycated haemoglobin, haemoglobin A1c or just A1c. It forms when haemoglobin joins with glucose in the blood. Your level of control will be measured by your health practitioner with these target ranges. Discuss with your healthcare professional to understand this fully. There are, however, a few occasions when HbA1c cannot be used for diagnosis and management of type 2 diabetes due to blood abnormality, and this has not been discussed in this book.

HbA1c ranges are shown in the table below.

HbA1c Category	HbA1c Range (Percentage)	HbA1c Range (mmol/mol)
Normal	Less than 6.0%	Less than 42 mmol/mol
Pre-diabetic	6.0% to 6.4%	42 to 47 mmol/mol
Diabetic	6.5% or higher	48 mmol/mol or higher

It's important to note that these ranges may vary slightly depending on the specific guidelines being used, and it's important to work with a healthcare professional to determine an appropriate HbA1c target range for your specific health needs and circumstances.

Interesting history!

Educate yourself. Become a sponge. There's so much information on diabetes out there. Diabetes Mellitus has been affecting lives for thousands of years. The origin of its name dates to around 230-250 BC. A Greek physician Apollonius of Memphis is credited with the given name "diabetes" meaning "to go through" due to its top symptom of excessive passing of urine through the body's system. Mellitus is a Latin word meaning honeyed or sweet. In the 17th century, diabetes was known as the "pissing evil."

Although the real cause of diabetes isn't fully understood, type 2 diabetes has been linked to being overweight or obese. The charity "Diabetes UK" states that being obese accounts for 80 to 85% of the risk of developing type 2 diabetes and rather than Body Mass Index (BMI >30kg/m2), central obesity (having a large waistline) is a better predictor of type 2 diabetes. Obesity is a medical condition in which the excess fat in the body has accumulated so much that it may have a negative effect on health.

Despite the link between excess weight and type 2 diabetes, there may be other factors driving this trend such as genetic mutations, a hormone not widely known called amylin (found in the pancreas), as well as disturbance in the body's natural clock.

Genetics is a big factor, as certain ethnic groups get type 2 diabetes at a much higher rate and at a much younger age. Diagnosis of type 2 diabetes is probably about 50% luck in the case of family history and 50% your lifestyle. Some slim people get type 2 diabetes and others, no matter their weight, won't get it. With all these differences, type 2 diabetes is thought to be polygenic.

Whatever these other factors are, weight is modifiable to help manage type 2 diabetes. Just by losing five to ten percent of your body weight can make a significant difference in managing type 2 diabetes.

Exploring our foods

How do you control diabetes by what you eat? Remember the saying, "you are what you eat." This is essentially true, though not completely. Diabetes as we mentioned earlier might have a hormonal as well as a genetic cause in addition to lifestyle. It's important to address changes that we can affect. For the majority of type 2 diabetes cases, modifying diets can be a game changer. The challenge is to decide to act and plan how this is going to happen. There are so many diets out there. What you choose should be what feels comfortable to you.

First, change your mindset. Feel and believe it when you say to yourself out loud, "I'm going to reverse my diabetes, no matter what it takes." "I'm going to control my diabetes, no matter what it takes." Keep saying it! Write it down! Journal about it every day! Put this statement up in prominent places in your home so that you can see it anytime you're walking past. For example, as you walk into the kitchen. You can use this as your phone background and your computer screen in your workspace. This helps when your other mind is trying to bring you back to your comfort zone. Practicing affirmations and continuously acting on them breed habits that eventually become second nature to you.

Change your environment by going round and pulling out all processed foods, sugary foods in the home. Sugary foods are really tempting and addicting. Get rid of them. Inform or discuss with your family or housemates living with you about your plan. They may decide to join you, encourage you, respect your wishes, or completely ignore you. This is where resilience kicks in. The support of people around you'll make it easier for you.

Now, what do you buy? Make a list of all the things you plan to eat for the whole week. Think of healthy alternative swaps. Don't rush this process. Consider buying healthy foods that you already like. Healthy eating is eating a wide variety of foods rich in nutrients in the right proportion, at the right time, and mindfully to achieve a weight that's healthy and balanced.

Here are few tips for eating healthily. Avoid skipping meals, as this may encourage snacking. Eat fruits and vegetable to reach five per day. Select different colours of fruit and vegetables to give a wider range of vitamins and minerals. Eat at least two portions of oily fish a week. Plant based proteins like beans, peas, and lentils are good and have little effect on blood glucose levels. They're a great source of protein and fibre and can improve good cholesterol levels. Wholegrain carbohydrates are preferred to refined grain carbohydrates as wholegrain (WG) contains the bran that's a great source of vitamin B, fibre, and minerals. Such examples are WG oats, WG porridge, WG bread, WG pasta, and brown rice. Reduce your sugar intake to not more than 30g a day. Cut down on sugary foods and drinks as this will help weight loss. Low fat dairy products are an option. Diary is important for bone and teeth health. Aim for 3 portions of dairy daily. You can have milk, a pot of yogurt, and a slice of cheese. Try to avoid foods heavy in saturated fats, foods heavy in trans fats, processed meats, sugary drinks, high-fat dairy products, salty foods, fried foods, and processed foods. Instead, choose healthy fat foods high in monosaturated fats such as avocado, olive oil, and nuts. Polyunsaturated fats like oily fish and seeds are encouraged. A healthy tip is to remove visible fat from meat and skin from chicken. You can also swap chocolate and crisps for nuts as a nutritious snack. Alcohol is high in calories. There have been extensive studies on the effect of alcohol on the body, some of which show contradictory results on improving or decreasing glucose tolerance (efficiency of the pancreas in effecting insulin production). Due the inconclusive nature of the studies, I will write in terms of weight loss. Having some alcohol-free days in a week is an effective way to cut back on calories that have little or no nutritional value and will result in weight loss. The National Health Service England recommend not more than 14 units of alcohol per week over several days. One unit is equivalent to 10ml or 8 grams of pure alcohol. This is about the average amount of alcohol an average adult can process in an hour and this will vary from person to person. It's easy to get confused about how many units there are in a drink, with so many different concentrations of drinks, bottles and glass sizes, pints, and shots. This idea of counting alcohol was introduced by the health service in 1987 to help people keep track of their alcohol consumption. You can look up the NHS website for more tips on calculating alcohol units. The recommendation is that diabetics should reduce significantly or stop alcohol consumption.

Reducing salt in your diet is a good habit to adapt, as high salt consumption can raise blood pressure and increase the risk of heart disease and stroke. An alternative way to flavour your dish when cooking is to use more herbs and spices.

There are so many dietary recommendations and dietary plans to choose from for weight loss. It's so easy to get overwhelmed and confused.

To briefly mention a few, there's the low-carbohydrate (low-carb) diet, the low-fat diet, the ketogenic diet (keto diet), the vegetarian diet, the vegan diets, the reducetarian diet or a version of the Mediterranean or DASH diet. I'll compare the low-carb and the low-fat diet.

Low carb vs low fat

There's been debates of low-carb vs. low-fat diets and which one is more effective for weight loss. The experts and media seem to constantly change their minds regarding this issue.

Low-fat diets have been popular since the 1980s and are still recommended for weight loss and to lower cholesterol to reduce risk of heart disease. Any fat is high in calories. One gram of fat will give 9 calories compared to one gram of carbohydrates or protein, which will give 4 calories. Lower fat intake will always result in weight loss in all age groups. It's important to recognise that in the process of sticking to this diet, you might be eliminating fatty acids, which helps to absorb the fat-soluble nutrients, vitamins, A, D, and E. Also, low-fat processed foods contain lots of sugar, which are high in calories and trick the buyer to consume more. A typical example applies in some fat-free yogurts.

The low-carb diet is a later occurrence in the weight-loss scene, which is popular. Some of these diets are the Atkins (at some stage, it was popular), Dukan, South Beach, and, more recently, ketogenic (keto) diets. Keto solicits eating a lot of meat, poultry, fish, eggs, and some non-starchy vegetables, but little to no grains (bread, pasta, rice and oats), legumes, fruit, and starchy vegetables. Some low-carb diet plans also limit nuts and seeds. Many low-carb diets boast of fast, effective weight loss and are often associated with health benefits of reducing the risk of type 2 diabetes and metabolic syndrome. Supporters believe the low-carb approach works because eating fewer carbs means you trigger the production of smaller amounts of the hormone insulin that causes the glucose your body absorbs from carbs to enter your body's cells. Since carbohydrates comprise the main source of energy for the body, reducing the amount consumed would make the body burn more of its stored fat required to work up energy, and this will lead to loss of weight. It's important to understand that not all carbohydrates are the same and that some, such as those found in fruits, vegetables, and whole grains, can be an important part of a healthy diet for people with diabetes. The American Diabetes Association (ADA) recommends that individuals with diabetes should aim to consume a personalized amount of carbohydrates based on their age, gender, weight, physical activity level, medication use, and blood glucose control. However, as a general guideline, the ADA suggests that people with diabetes should aim for around 45-60 grams of carbohydrates per meal, which would equate to approximately 135-180 grams of carbohydrates per day across three meals. Keep in mind that these are just general recommendations, and the amount of carbohydrates that an individual needs may vary based on their individual needs and goals.

In recent years, there has been a lot of debate about the best type of diet for weight loss and overall health. The two popular types of diets that are often compared are low-fat and low-carb diets. Low-fat diets have traditionally been recommended to reduce the risk of heart disease and other chronic illnesses, while low-carb diets have gained popularity for their potential to aid in weight loss.

However, studies in recent years have shown that there may not be as much of a difference between the two types of diets as previously thought. For example, a study by

Gardner et al. published in the *Journal of the American Medical Association* in 2018 compared the effects of a low-fat diet to a low-carb diet on weight loss and found that there was no significant difference between the two diets in terms of weight loss or improvements in cardiovascular risk factors.

Another study published in The Lancet in 2018 compared the effects of a low-fat diet, a low-carb diet, and a moderate carb diet on weight loss and found that all three diets led to similar weight loss after 12 months. Additionally, there was no significant difference between the diets in terms of changes in blood pressure, cholesterol levels, or other health markers.

While these studies suggest that there may not be a significant difference between low-fat and low-carb diets, it's important to note that our response to different types of diets can vary. Some people may find that they do better on a low-fat diet, while others may do better on a low-carb diet. It's also worth noting that the quality of the food consumed is just as important as the macronutrient composition of the diet. A diet that consists of highly processed foods, regardless of its fat or carb content, is unlikely to be beneficial to health.

Proteins are important and required by the body for various functions such as building and repairing tissues, making enzymes, hormones, and other body chemicals. However, when the body is lacking in carbohydrates and fats, it can use proteins as an alternative source of energy. This process is known as gluconeogenesis, which is the breakdown of proteins to produce glucose for energy.

While the body can use proteins as an energy source, this can have negative effects on the body. One of the most significant effects is the loss of muscle mass, which can ultimately lead to a decrease in overall body mass.

Another potential negative effect of using proteins as an energy source is the impact on the immune system. Proteins are essential for building and maintaining a healthy immune system. However, when the body is using proteins for energy, it can reduce the amount of available proteins for immune system function. This can weaken the immune system and increase the risk of infections and other illnesses.

In addition, using proteins as an energy source can also lead to other negative effects such as fatigue, weakness, and nutrient deficiencies. This is because the body needs a balanced intake of carbohydrates, proteins, and fats to function optimally.

Therefore, it is important to consume an adequate amount of carbohydrates and fats to prevent the body from using proteins as an energy source and to maintain optimal body mass and immune system function. Cutting out carbohydrates can deny you of the positive nutrients obtained from carbohydrates in the long run. Also, cutting carbs means eating more saturated fats which can lead to increased cholesterol and heart disease. The short-term side effects are headaches, weakness, nausea, dizziness, and irritability when your body breaks down stored fat to produce energy, producing ketones. The question is whether a strict keto diet is sustainable in the long term.

Reference calories

The recommended calorie intake for women is 2,000 calories and men 2,500 calories a day! With diabetes, you can reduce your calorie intake with a controlled meal plan. The U.S Department of Agriculture (USDA) website has daily nutrient recommendations based on the Dietary Reference Intakes (DRIs) by age and by gender. Accessing this website, takes you to myplateplan.gov website which gives you a nutritional guide to healthy food options describing how much and what to eat within your calorie allowance. You may want to visit your healthcare professional who can refer you to a diabetic educational class. Other options are finding a dietitian with diabetic knowledge to tailor your diet to suit you, looking up reliable diets online, or, better still, designing your own diet based on your research. If one diet plan doesn't work, pick up yourself and try another. Growth is a continuous process and we have to keep learning and changing in the right direction.

Here are a few examples of books that may give information and guidance on managing diabetes through diet.

The Diabetes Code: *Prevent and Reverse Type 2 Diabetes Naturally* by Dr Jason Fung - This book provides an in-depth look at the causes and management of type 2 diabetes through diet and lifestyle changes.

The Complete Diabetic Cookbook: *Delicious and Balanced Recipes Made Easy* by America's Test Kitchen - This cookbook provides a collection of easy-to-follow recipes that are specifically designed for people with diabetes. The recipes are balanced, nutritious, and delicious.

The Low-Carb Diabetes Solution Cookbook: *Prevent and Heal Type 2 Diabetes with 200 Ultra Low-Carb Recipes* by Dana Carpender - This cookbook provides a collection of ultra-low-carb recipes that are specifically designed for people with diabetes. The recipes are easy to make and use simple, affordable ingredients.

The Mediterranean Diabetes Cookbook by Amy Riolo - This cookbook provides a collection of Mediterranean-inspired recipes that are specifically designed for people with diabetes. The recipes are delicious and use fresh, whole ingredients.

The Ultimate Guide to Accurate Carb Counting: *Featuring the Tools and Techniques Used by the Experts* by Gary Scheiner - This book provides a comprehensive guide to counting carbohydrates and managing diabetes through diet. It includes tips, tools, and techniques used by diabetes experts to manage blood sugar levels.

Although these books can provide helpful guidance and information, it's always best to consult with your healthcare professional or a registered diabetic dietitian to tailor your dietary plan to your individual needs.

Pharmacists and other health professionals familiar within this space, are aware that there's no one size fits all when it comes to helping people lose weight and leading a healthier lifestyle to kick overweight and improve sugar levels in the blood. Weight loss plans should be tailored to the individual, where they find a process, they can enjoy and stick to long term, and not a quick fix diet that they'll eventually give up on. It's obvious that many get confused and misled with all the information out there. We have the duty to cut through these dieting trends as they're unlikely to cease and support such individuals in their health journeys in whatever healthy eating plan they feel is right for them. Please contact your healthcare practitioner who can direct you to accredited programs in your area.

Intermittent fasting

The Physician Within: ***"Everyone has a physician inside him or her; we just have to help it in its work. The natural healing force within each one of us is the greatest force in getting well. Our food should be our medicine. Our medicine should be our food. But to eat when you are sick is to feed your sickness."*** —Hippocrates

Fasting exists in many religious practices and it is defined in the Free dictionary as "voluntarily not eating food for varying lengths of time." The abstention will usually involve some or all kinds of food and/or drink for a period. You might want to learn a bit of history! The Ancient Greeks greatly believed in fasting, and fasting is said to have originated in Greece and dates to 460 BC. Pythagoras and Hippocrates were on the forefront of fasting. Pythagoras created the Pythagorean theorem in maths and at the time was known to go without food for up to forty days at a time to improve creativity and mental insight. He was vegetarian when he ate, and the same applied to his followers who were called the Pythagoreans. Similarly, Hippocrates, who was a physician, was called by some as the Father of Medicine. He formed the Hippocratic food of Medicine and is recognised for the Mediterranean diet which has the whole package diet where you drink some wine, yogurt, cheese, vegetable, fish, fruits, whole cereals, legumes, and use olive oil all in appropriate portions. In our current world, the Mediterranean diet is linked to longevity, positively affecting the brain and the heart. It's a highly recommended diet in type 2 diabetes. The opening quote at beginning of this chapter is said to be Hippocrates's quote on fasting. It emphasises the importance of fasting during illness or disease. Hippocrates, who is considered the father of Western medicine, believed that fasting could promote healing by allowing the body's natural healing mechanisms to work more effectively.

Intermittent fasting (IF) is an eating pattern where one can individually go without eating for a set period. Intermittent fasting (or intermittent energy restriction) is also described as when there's a restriction of any of the mealtime schedules that could cycle between voluntary fasting (or calorie restriction) and non-fasting over a given period. The advantage of IF is than it doesn't depend on any diet plan. When done right, it could produce great therapeutic results. This isn't an encouraging statement to throw your healthy eating plan to the wind. If you decide after reading about IF to try it out, you must keep to your healthy eating plan. The different IF types include daily time-restricted fasting (16:8 - is quite popular, where you fast for 16 hours and eat in the 8-hour window), the periodic fasting and the alternate-day fasting (5:2 - 2 days of fasting in the week, either zero calorie on the 2 days a week or modified to consume 500 calories only on 2 days of the week). The restriction or reduction of calorie intake that's not detrimental to health is promising and thought of as a dietary intervention that could extend the lifespan of humans. To continuously reduce calorie intake in an overweight or obese patient isn't as easy as it sounds in real-live situations. Fasting interventions and feeding restricted by time have emerged as substitutes or possibilities.

Patikorn et al. (2021) investigated the impact of IF on health outcomes related to obesity and discovered notable connections between weight loss and cardiometabolic health, particularly with the modified alternate day fasting approach. This approach involves consuming only 500 calories on fasting days and maintaining a regular, healthy diet on the other five days. More clinical trials are needed for long-term clinical outcomes for preventing cardiovascular events and mortality. This is possibly one of the reasons why clinicians are cautious in recommending IF due to the lack of evidence on the long-term benefits. IF certainly has not been studied in children, the elderly, and underweight individuals, and I would advise against these categories. It's recommended you discuss with your healthcare professional before commencing intermittent fasting if you belong in the above-mentioned categories. Using IF for glucose and weight control is rapidly emerging and only time will give it the boost it probably deserves.

There are other possible benefits like the 2021 study by Gudden and his research team who discussed the positive effects IF may have on the brain and on cognitive function, and observed how the variation in the fasting patterns and total calorie intake may contribute towards its success.

In another study published in 2014 by *The Journal of Cell Metabolism*, we also see how prolonged overnight fasting could extend healthy lifespan by promoting autophagy. Autophagy is a natural degradation and removal and recycling of unnecessary or dysfunctional cell components through a regulated mechanism by the body. Fruit flies were used in this experiment, which explored the effects of intermittent fasting on autophagy in fruit flies. The study used genetic methods to block autophagy in the fruit flies and found that those who were unable to undergo autophagy did not experience the same benefits from intermittent fasting as those who could undergo autophagy. Specifically, the flies that were able to undergo autophagy showed increased lifespan, improved motor function, and decreased accumulation of toxic proteins compared to the flies that could not undergo autophagy. The study suggests that autophagy is an important process that contributes to the health benefits of intermittent fasting. Although the molecular mechanisms are unclear, the study highlighted the beneficial possibility that a change in behaviour to stimulate a circadian regulated autophagy could delay ageing and prolong life. This little bit of information if nothing else, should discourage us from night-time snacking and to stop eating as early as we can for the day.

Story: Forty-five-year-old John who had been diabetic for 2 years was struggling with his weight, and blood sugar levels were creeping up. He had tried many diets, but nothing seemed to work for him. One day, a friend introduced him to the concept of intermittent fasting. At first, he was sceptical, but decided to give it a try.

To his surprise, he found that intermittent fasting was much easier to stick to than other diets he had tried. By eating within a certain time frame, he was able to control his portion sizes and make healthier food choices. He also found that he had more energy and focus throughout the day.

As a result of intermittent fasting, John lost weight, improved his blood sugar levels, and lowered his risk of heart disease. He was so pleased with the results that he started to recommend intermittent fasting to others.

Intermittent fasting in John's eyes can be a powerful tool for improving health and achieving weight loss goals. It's important to consult with a healthcare professional before starting any new diet."

Water, the basic idea!

Drinking water sits in the centre of a healthy lifestyle. There's no secret to its importance in our overall health. We need water for our basic survival. In this chapter, I'll focus on why diabetics need to drink more water. Simply increasing your water intake can give great benefits. Generally, whether you're diabetic or not, most of us should be drinking a little more water. Each cell and organ in our bodies need water to function normally, and water helps get rid of waste products in the system. There are varying recommendations on how much to drink daily: some say two litres while others say eight cups. These are all rough estimates, and drinking when thirsty should give similar results. A number of factors could affect the amount of water that's consumed and can depend on activity levels, ambient temperature, body size, and whether you are male or female, as males need to drink more water than females.

Try observing how much you drink daily. Is it more or less than 2 litres? Do you have to drink more?

Water helps lower blood sugar levels. When your blood sugar levels are high, the kidneys attempt to excrete excess sugar from the body. Increasing water intake will help the kidneys facilitate the process of excretion of excess glucose which is passed out as urine. Hyperglycaemia can lead to dehydration due to concentrated glucose in the blood stream. Typical symptoms of dehydration are headache, dizziness, fatigue, dark urine, and a strong urine smell. Also, drinking sufficient water is a great way to stay in remission from diabetes.

Generally, we all know that water aids digestion; in addition, it improves liver health, clears the complexion of the skin, and gives a youthful look, prolonging the onset of wrinkles. Water breaks the snacking habit, as, sometimes, we think we're hungry when what we really need is a drink of water. Try substituting water or a low glycaemic drink for one of your snacks and see how you feel. This is one great way to lose weight.

It's normal to want a change from plain water sometimes. Here are some tips to spicing up your drink without affecting your glycaemic levels. Drinks like sparkling water and soda water are some alternatives. You can become innovative by squeezing in lemon or lime or brewing some of your favourite herbs.

Story: Preeti, 47 years of age had been struggling with managing her diabetes for 6 years. She tried improving her diet and different treatments, but there was little improvement. One day, her nurse suggested that she consciously try drinking more water, as it could help regulate her blood sugar levels.

At first, Preeti was sceptical, but she was desperate for anything that could help improve her condition, so she decided to give it a try. To her surprise, Preeti noticed a significant difference in just a few days. The more water she drank, the more stable her blood sugar levels became.

Encouraged by her success, Preeti started to research the relationship between water and diabetes management. She learned that water helps flush out excess glucose from the body, which is a major contributing factor to high blood sugar levels. It also helps the body absorb insulin more effectively, which is essential for managing diabetes.

Preeti continued to drink plenty of water every day, and her diabetes management improved dramatically. She no longer had to worry about sudden spikes or drops in her blood sugar levels, and she was able to enjoy a much better quality of life.

Preeti makes sure she drinks plenty of water every day, and she remembers how a simple change in her habits had made such a huge impact on her life. She became a passionate advocate for the benefits of drinking water, and inspired others to make the same change.

Moving

Keep moving, don't stay still. Exercise plays an important role in type 2 diabetes. It can lower blood sugar levels, insulin requirements, and stress levels. American Diabetes Association (ADA) recommends not to miss aerobic exercises more than twice in a row. Current ADA guidelines recommend aerobic, resistance, and combined exercises for the management of type 2 diabetes. According to the National Institutes of Health (NIH), at least 150 minutes of moderate-intensity aerobic exercise spread over a minimum of three days per week is recommended for adults with diabetes, and with no more than two consecutive days without exercise. Also, strength training exercises at least two days per week, targeting all major muscle groups is recommended. Sue Cotey and Andrea Harris, diabetes specialists from the Cleveland clinic recommend some general exercises that are easy to fit into your normal daily activities such as walking, Tai Chi, yoga, and dancing.

Walking is the most popular and the most easily achievable form of exercise as can be done anywhere. Thirty minutes of brisk walking, five times a week is a good way to increase physical activity. This can also be broken down into three ten-minute walks a day.

Tai Chi is from Chinese origin, sometimes colloquially known as "shadowboxing." Wikipedia describes Tai Chi as an internal Chinese martial art usually practiced for defence training, health benefits, and meditation. It combines deep breathing and relaxation with flowing movements. Check out the nhs.uk/live-well/exercise/guide-to-tai-chi for more information on Tai Chi. Studies have shown significant improvement in blood sugar control, and students of Tai Chi report increased vitality, energy, and mental health.

Yoga is a traditional form of exercise that builds on balance, strength, and flexibility. It can lower stress and improve nerve function, resulting in increased wellness and improved blood glucose due to improved muscle mass, according to the ADA.

Dancing can also be a great form of exercise. Trying to remember dance steps improves your brain power and memory. In diabetes, it can make increasing physical activity fun and hence promote weight loss, improve flexibility, lower blood glucose, and help with stress reduction. In 30 minutes of active dance, a 150-pound adult can burn up to 150 calories.

Swimming is a good form of activity for all including diabetics, as it stretches and relaxes your muscles without feeling the pressure on your joints. Swimming can improve the levels of cholesterol in your body, burn calories, and lower levels of stress, and it may improve depression-like behaviour. Swimming can gradually be built up. Always inform the lifeguard that you have diabetes before getting into the pool.

Safety tips: Build up your exercise gradually, especially if you're new to a selected regimen or haven't been active for a while. Start slowly, avoid high-intensity and heavy lifting initially, then build up if you can. Speak to your doctor or healthcare professional to be sure your choice of exercise is right for you and report any unusual effects. More importantly, listen to your body. Know how your body works; check blood sugar before and after exercise. Drink lots of water before, during, and after exercise to keep rehydrated. Be prepared for hypoglycaemia (low blood glucose) and have something to increase sugar levels such as glucose tablets, sugary juice. Try eating snacks high in protein before a workout to sustain you at a normal glucose level as you exercise. Always carry a mobile phone to use in case you need to call for help. Exercise in mild conditions; avoid extreme temperatures. Wear appropriate footwear and socks to protect your feet.

The 7 mindsets

I came across the 7 mindsets, a social emotional learning style that resonates with me. There have been extensive studies on social emotional learning, and its positive solution is based on ground-breaking research. Although, adapted for use in schools for children and educationalists, I am confident it could be applied to diabetes to help recondition the mind to think positively. I'll take you through the 7 mindsets of positivity.

1. Everything is possible - When nothing is certain, everything is possible. This mindset is the positive power of dreaming big and maintaining positive expectations. A positive mindset makes dreams a reality. It's the belief that through determination and hard work, you can send your diabetes into remission or have tight control over your blood glucose to eliminate the worry or stress that comes with it. Be creative and imaginative, read books on health, listen to podcasts, talk to a friend. These can expand your mind to greater awareness. You become happier with the possibility of a better future. Action brings success. Our greatest obstacle to taking action is fear of failure. Remember, this is your own journey; there's no comparing with anyone. There's no failure. You learn from your mistakes and move on. Act and adjust.

2. Passion first - People with great passion can make the impossible happen. You need to connect your passion to what you really want to achieve and your pursuits of making maximum progress. What's your individual genius? What are you good at? What do you like doing?

What are your strengths? This should help in what form of exercise you choose to take on, modify, or improve to increase your physical activity. It's like taking up tennis when the best thing you can think of is hitting a tennis ball. Focus on your strengths. Do more of walking if you like walking. You can increase your steps daily, weekly, or monthly. You can be the first person who put their diabetes into remission through walking in your group or can join an inspiring group of individuals who have achieved great things and served as positive role models for others with type 2 diabetes. Some examples of such individuals are Tom Hanks - the Academy Award-winning actor who was diagnosed with type 2 diabetes in 2013. Tom has been open about his diagnosis and he has spoken about the importance of managing the condition through diet and exercise. Sherri Shepherd, a comedian and actress was diagnosed with type 2 diabetes in 2007. She has since become an advocate for diabetes awareness and has spoken publicly about her struggles with the condition. Then DJ Spinderella, the legendary hip-hop DJ and producer was diagnosed with type 2 diabetes in 2009. She has lost over 50 pounds through diet and exercise and has become an advocate for healthy living and diabetes awareness.

This shows that it's possible to live a healthy and fulfilling life with type 2 diabetes, and that with proper management, diabetes doesn't have to hold you back from achieving your goals.

Understand your core values, as you'll always go back to this during trying and challenging times. Be authentic with yourself, as this will drive passion and help fulfil your dreams.

3. We are all connected - No one is an island. This explores the synergies in relationships. In the course of diagnosis of type 2 diabetes, you've met new people, medical personnel, administration staff, other people with similar conditions, and visited places you wouldn't have ordinarily gone. You also have people in your life before diabetes diagnosis. This realisation allows us to understand that people who come into our lives can help us achieve our goals and shows the importance of exploring synergies. People you meet in your life have the potential to help you, hurt you, or have no impact at all. To ensure that you're making progress towards your goals, it's wise to assess how each individual can assist you, as choosing alternative options may not lead you any closer to achieving them. Living a great live might mean embracing everyone and constantly looking for ways to serve and be served by people you encounter. However, maximise the positive relationships, as these people will lift you up, encourage you, and make you better. You may like to join diabetes forums where you hear other people's stories and learn from those who've been living with diabetes and who have experiences you can draw from. Unfortunately, there are people who can bring you down, but you have the choice to spend less time with such people. An important step is to recognise the critical role people can play in your life and to develop relationships with the positive ones. Lead with value when you find people who can help you. You can start creating mutually beneficial relationships quickly so that the cycle of giving can begin. Many have learned that if you offer help before you ask for help, you're almost certain to get more out of the relationship.

4. 100% accountability - "At the end of the day, we're accountable to ourselves – our success is a result of what we do." —Catherine Pulsifer. (*"Personal accountability, requires mindfulness, acceptance, honesty and courage." —Shelby Martin).* It's your choice to be responsible for your own health and well-being. This mindset teaches us that we're not victims of our past, our future isn't predetermined, and our lives are what we choose. It enables us to recognise our fears and the excuses we make, helps to break down barriers, to free our minds and then focus our energy to take the important steps towards our goals. Own all aspects of your life and be free to act and think for yourself. Your friendships might change in situations when you decide to cut down on your regular pub visits every Friday with friends or colleagues to avoid alcohol. Don't allow others to control your life.

Overcome limiting beliefs. You are limitless, and it is possible! Limitations we place on ourselves present in form of fear, excuses, and counter mindsets. Your way of thinking can be reprogrammed to overpower limiting beliefs. Use your energy to learn and accomplish what's important to you to get the most out of each day. Learn from all experiences and get better. If one diet or exercise doesn't suit you, pick yourself up and try another. Doing this will make you accountable.

5. Attitude of gratitude - we look for the positives in every experience by having an attitude of gratitude mindset and being thankful for all we have. As individuals, we can either choose the positives or the negatives to build our foundation in life. We can go on a tangent of why me, which can worsen the situation or choose the positive as that of gratitude which can lead to a brilliant success in effecting change. Gratitude involves focusing on what we have and not being distracted by what we don't have. We might have diabetes, but we must recognise the treasure in us, cherish and grow this to enable you to live a great life. Focusing on anger, blame, or regret can increase your negative experience. Be more grateful as often as you can. Think of good things in your life.

One of the ways to feel better and happier is by service, by doing something for another person. You can affect someone's mood by expressing gratitude for who they or what they have done for you. It makes the other person feel good and gives you good feelings in the process. Expand Your Perspective. People who have had success in what they have done would describe moments of difficulty or challenges as important lessons in developing essential skills that allowed them to be successful. Gratitude is such a strong practice that yields the advantages of being thankful for now and seeing the positives in the negatives. By managing your diabetes through healthy eating and exercise, you can reduce the risk of developing other chronic health conditions such as heart disease, stroke, and high blood pressure, and you can become an advocate for diabetes awareness and education, sharing your experience and helping others manage their condition, thus allowing you to live a richer life by essentially learning and growing.

6. Live to give - Make positive differences in the lives of others and build symbiotic relationships. You can use one little step at success in your diabetic control to inspire and serve others while you're still on your own journey to remission or tight control of your condition. Live to give describes abundance in one's life as a cycle, and to get love, respect, and financial security, we must learn to give the same. It doesn't necessarily have to be in the same area of experience. For example, during an online educational program, you might notice that a person is struggling to grasp the technicalities of operating or manoeuvring the course content. You can offer to show/teach them an easy way to operate and in exchange, they can give you tips on how they've managed to cross a different hurdle that you seem stuck on, such as limiting your calorie consumption for breakfast. In other words, use your unique genius to make positive impacts, knowing that good things will return to you in kind. It's right to be of service, and the best way to get what you want is to give what you can. Here, both parties gain, including others around you. When you start giving, you become happier. Start making a little difference every day and this will create value in your life. Receive gracefully, no matter how uncomfortable it feels, to continue the cycle, as these spur you on to keep giving and prevent you from limiting your own potential. Leave a legacy that will impact others and the world to make your life transcend you.

7. The time is now - Make every moment count. Live in the present. What can we do now to effect a change in the future that eventually becomes our now? How willing are we to take a decisive positive step to leave a healthy happier life? All our power exists in the moment; the past is gone, we cannot change it, and the future is yet to come. Why not take a determined action in the present to create a better tomorrow? Embrace every moment. How is your healthy eating going? Did you lose 1 pound in 2 weeks? Celebrate your positive emotions. No matter how little, celebrate, as this encourages you to do more. You can also change a negative emotion to a positive through acceptance then devising methods to change for the better. Acting in anger or confusion can often cause a wrong action. It can ultimately make you abandon your lifestyle plan and go back to square one. Try to recognise this and stop! Find a way to get into a better state of mind. Once you're in your zone, the actions taken would be more effective and give a more positive result. Think before you act!

It okay to be vulnerable; in this state, your emotions are quite intense. You might have gone out with a friend and couldn't resist the temptation of a burger, fries, and cheesecake with caramel fudge sauce, and now you feel so guilty about it. You're upset. It's important to recognise that setbacks happen and that you can restart. You might have a community group you can talk to, an accountability partner, or even your healthcare professional. These groups or people are usually supportive and nonjudgemental, and it's easier to pick yourself up and start again. Don't be surprised if you encounter a similar situation with someone in the group and notice how the responses from the group will pick you up again.

Act on purpose - always remember your values. Actions taken will be yours because they resonate with you and matter to you. Your purpose would push you to try harder, knowing what the goal is. The steps you're taking to achieve need to be regularly reviewed, and always ask: Is the action I'm taking moving me towards the life I want?

Chapter 4: Understanding Mindfulness

"The mind is just like a muscle - the more you exercise it, the stronger it gets and the more it can expand." —Idowu Koyenikan

Mindfulness and meditation

Meditation and mindfulness are used interchangeably often. These two words have been used a lot in modern times as people search for calm and inner peace in their daily lives. Both are interrelated but not the same. Mindfulness is based on Zen Buddhism which lies in the ancient practice of meditation. Mindfulness has become so popular that it's embedded in our everyday language. It encourages conscious awareness of whatever our focus might be, encouraging us to take good care of ourselves. As such, anybody can practice, irrespective of culture or religion.

Walsh and Shapiro described meditation as a practice where an individual uses a technique, such as mindfulness or focusing the mind on a particular object, thought, or activity, to train attention and awareness and achieve a mentally clear and emotionally calm and stable state.

John Kabat-Zinn, the creator of Mindfulness-Based Stress Reduction program (MBSR), defined mindfulness as paying conscious attention to the present moment, on purpose and being non-judgemental to what you're experiencing.

I draw from these definitions that meditation is a practice, and one can, through this practice, develop different qualities, including mindfulness. Mindfulness is a form of meditation, and it relates to a specific way of living that can be refined through practice. One way one can learn to live mindfully is through meditation. Living mindfully involves cultivating a habit of paying attention to the present, moment-by-moment thoughts, emotions, and physical sensations with openness, curiosity, and non-judgemental awareness. With regular practice, you can learn to live each moment more fully and with greater ease and clarity. Overall, mindfulness and meditation are closely related, and practicing mindfulness meditation can be an effective way to learn to live mindfully.

It can help you cope in difficult times and improve your mental state and physical wellbeing. It can break down that cycle of stress and anxiety, as well as depression.

There are other ways to live mindfully without using meditation, as some people aren't receptive to the word "meditation." According to Thompson and Walz (2015), mindfulness has been associated with many health benefits and positive qualities such as self-esteem and self-acceptance.

The practice of mindfulness is familiar to me, and there seems to be more to learn every day, in reaping the benefits of calmness and clarity. We as humans have the ability to tailor practices to suit our needs. It's rewarding to experience calm in situations that one would normally find challenging and spend time worrying. Daily meditative practice helps bring that inner peace and decrease negative thoughts. Now my mantra is: "Why worry about yesterday or tomorrow, how about now, being present in this very moment?" I try to be present regularly in stolen moments of my busy schedule and this helps to recentre me. With my experience in clinical practice and consulting with patients with diabetes, I feel certain mindful practices in different aspects of our lives can be beneficial. Mindfulness is a call to observe your thoughts but not to avoid them. It addresses the mental turmoil when diagnosed with or when managing diabetes. There's nothing wrong with accepting the way you're feeling rather than always resisting and trying to change it. By accepting first, you can then think of the best approach of change. There are different ways to practice mindfulness. Practice could be guided by a trained person with you as the only participant or in a group. You can also use other resources like a mindfulness book, an app, or in podcasts.

Dialectical behaviour therapy (DBT) is a treatment example that uses mindfulness practice to help people without requiring formal meditation. The aim is to help the person to develop a "wise mind" (a balance between the reasonable mind and the emotional mind) by learning different skills that helps them live mindfully. Benjamin Shapero, a clinical psychologist, and his team explored mindfulness based cognitive therapy in treating depression and studies show that it may improve psychological health. Clinicians can usually guide their clients towards mindfulness, and they won't have to become involved in a formal practice. It's good for when time is limited or there's hesitation by the individual. Mindfulness can be a formal or informal practice.

Meditation can be conflicting, as it's an exercise of "a lack of effort" as we're encouraged to become an observer of our mind, using minimal effort and observing without judgement. It's conflicting because most of us would not live our lives this way; instead, we're so busy prioritising work over rest. Usually, when we practice formal meditation, we sit for a planned period. This however makes us stop to think and remind us that we don't need to hammer away nonstop to achieve our goals or be who we want to be. This is formal mindfulness. Many people might not want to engage formally in mindful practice but will still want a daily mindfulness routine. Mindfulness is a call to accept before change and to engage rather than escape. This practice enables us to refresh our aim and remember our intention.

Mindfulness can be practiced in many informal ways, and it's encouraging to know that some of these informal mindful practices have beneficial effects on type 2 diabetes and other associated health conditions such as better sleep, better blood glucose levels, and much more. Such mindful practices include mindful eating, mindful breathing, mindful walking, and mindful conversations. Informal mindfulness practice means to participate in everyday activities with the intent of being mindful. It's a natural quality that we all have. We can simply become more aware of where we are and what we're doing with less reaction or without being overwhelmed by what's going on around us. It can alleviate stress, provide clarity, and promote peace of mind. It will enable you to plan and achieve your desired target, be it sending diabetes into remission or getting a tight control of type 2 diabetes. Whatever you practice in the mind grows stronger.

Hyperglycaemia is when the blood glucose levels are high. As there are slight variations in values depending on the country, the UK values for hyperglycaemia are 7mmol/l when fasting, or above 11.1 mmol/l at any time during the day. This can be problematic in type 2 diabetics and can lead to more long-term complications associated with diabetes such as raised blood pressure, heart attack, and stroke as mentioned earlier.

Hypoglycaemia, when the blood glucose levels are low, below 4mmol/l, is less common in type 2 diabetes and would usually occur due to dietary decisions, being on a certain medication, or if on insulin. Research has shown that mindfulness can improve glycaemic control, decreases episodes of hyperglycaemia or hypoglycaemia, leading a reduction in mental stress and depression associated with the management of diabetes.

How do we learn mindfulness? Mindfulness is a skill that can be developed with practice. Its attention can change the impact of and response to thoughts, feelings, and sensations. Mindfulness is process oriented rather than outcome driven.

It can be learned by just quietening the mind and being present wherever you are. You can practice what you've learnt in this book so far, attend an informal mindfulness or meditation class, or access other online mindfulness programmes. I found guided meditation quite grounding for me, especially at the initial stages of practice. Now I can practice mindfulness on my own or be guided in a group. The more you practice, the more beneficial it becomes. Mindfulness can also be practiced through taking part in clinical programs like Mindfulness- Based Stress Reduction classes or Mindfulness-Based Cognitive Therapy classes. Some online programmes on mindful practices could be of help. Mindfulness can be eclectic, as you can select different elements to design your own practice to suit your individual goals. Once this is discovered, you'll have to be patient; most importantly, be consistent in your routine and intentional about your goal. It takes time to form a habit, but once formed you'll experience the daily benefits of mindful practice.

Type 2 diabetes can be overwhelming! That's an understatement! Many people experience shock at the news that they've been diagnosed with diabetes following a blood test, even though a family member already has it. They're emotional and think, *Surely, it's a mistake. Let's redo the blood test.* The mind begins to race and thoughts of cutting out all kinds of junk food, giving up favourite meals, the sudden realisation that this is real, and it's not going away unless I change. Life is so busy; how do I get more time to look after myself? I must or face the consequences of prolonged denial. This was an exact rant by one of my patients. This is a worry and could cause depressive moods.

There are certain emotional stages we go through before accepting that diabetes is real and decide to fully embrace it and work positively towards controlling it. Kubler-Ross, a psychologist who discussed the theory of the stages of grief, explained the five stages: shock and denial; anger, frustration, and shame; depressed or detached; bargaining or dialogue; and, finally, acceptance. The theory always begins with the shock and denial phase when you cling to a false sense of reality. Then the anger phase, when you feel frustrated, irritable, anxious, embarrassed, or ashamed. You can then feel depressed and detached with lack or energy or overwhelm. The next stage is the bargaining or dialogue. Here, you might reach out to tell your story or try to find meaning to the cause of your condition. You finally get to the acceptance stage when you become willing to find solutions and put new plans in place because you've acceptable this as your true reality. The last stage occurs when life becomes more meaningful. You're empowered, secure, and your self-esteem is back. These stages may not necessarily happen in this fashion. It might be that some stages are skipped or happen so quickly that they're barely noticeable. I'm writing this for you to be aware that it's normal to experience the way you feel in a condition that you wished was never there. You may be one to go straight from acceptance to empowerment. For more information on the stages of the acceptance cycle, you can check online.

You may use mindfulness to overcome significant barriers that prevent effective self-management. We now know that both anxiety and depression can cause elevated levels of blood glucose; thus, it's expected that by practicing mindfulness, self-management will be improved naturally as psychological well-being increases.

We can summarise two basic ways in which mindfulness may help people control diabetes. First, it may directly help them to self-manage their diabetes. As they become more mindful, they're more present and in touch with their health needs from moment to moment. They have an increased awareness and clarity in thought and can make better decisions without judgement. Secondly, it can improve physical health, allowing them to enjoy their workout, knowing it's something they've chosen to do from their inner being.

Story: "David, a 46-year-old man had been living with type 2 diabetes for 5 years. He had tried everything to manage his condition, but nothing seemed to work. He felt like he was in a constant battle with his blood sugar levels and was always worried about the long-term complications of diabetes.

One day, a friend suggested that he try incorporating mindfulness into his diabetes management routine. David was hesitant at first but decided to give it a try. He started practicing mindfulness techniques such as deep breathing and meditation. He also started to focus on being present in the moment and paying attention to his thoughts and feelings.

Over time, David found that mindfulness helped him to better manage his diabetes. He found that he was more aware of his body and his feelings, which made it easier for him to make healthy choices. He also found that he was less stressed and more at peace with his condition.

David's story shows that mindfulness can be a powerful tool for managing type 2 diabetes. It can help to reduce stress, improve awareness, and make it easier to make healthy choices. Mindfulness can be a great addition to a diabetes management routine and can help improve overall health and well-being."

Depression and anxiety in type 2 diabetes

Mental healthcare is an integral part of diabetes management. Once diagnosed with diabetes, most thoughts seem to change automatically. We start to think of blood glucose levels with every meal we eat, keeping active, meal planning, and other things we've been advised by healthcare practitioners to do, read, or to avoid, and mostly what could happen if no action is taken. We go into thought overload. Thinking about all these can drain us emotionally and leave us completely overwhelmed, as it becomes too much to take in. We can term this "Diabetes Burnout," the overwhelming thoughts about how to cope. Always evaluate the way you feel. Ask yourself. How am I? Am I stressed, angry, sad, or scared of not coping? Remember that there's always help. Would it be helpful to speak to someone about how you're feeling, to improve your understanding, and develop strategies? Diabetes can impact mental health or mental health can impact diabetes. A great advice will be to ask your doctor to refer you to a reputable mental healthcare provider, therapist, or psychologist. Free self-referral to clinics are available in some countries like the UK, provided by the National Health Service (NHS). Remember that it's normal and expected to feel the way you're feeling.

There's some evidence that mindfulness can alleviate depression and anxiety. Some people with diabetes will often think of the carbohydrates in their diets, the way different foods release different amounts of glucose that will spark an increase in blood glucose levels, or the lifestyle decisions that must be made. This might include refusing an evening meal out with friends to avoid being tempted by the expanse of food choices at a time when you're focused on healthy eating. If you're on insulin, it's even more complex, checking blood sugar levels and injecting the right amount. This line of thought is just on food worries alone. It's no wonder many people with diabetes become anxious and depressed when other everyday processes that need addressing are also considered.

In anxiety and depression, you worry and ruminate. Worry usually focuses on thoughts of imagining future catastrophes that would rarely, if ever, actually occur, and it's often accompanied by a plan of what to do should they happen. Rumination, on the other hand, focuses on the past when there's continual reflection on imagined failings and how because of this, life is unlikely to improve. These obstructive ways of thinking would maintain anxiety and depression according to psychologists, which can be significant barriers to managing diabetes. Being able to focus on the here and now and change the thought and feeling process can give the opportunity to devote more time and energy into looking after ourselves.

Sleep

"True silence is the rest of the mind and is to the spirit what sleep is to the body, nourishment and refreshment." —William Penn

A lot of us don't appreciate sleep as much as we should. Insufficient or irregular sleep along with waking frequently during night sleep can cause insulin resistance. Nanna Lindekilde, affiliated with the psychology department of the University of Southern Denmark, conducted a study in 2016 revealing that sleep disorders have a significant impact on blood glucose levels and may contribute to the development of type 2 diabetes. According to other researchers, there is a bidirectional relationship between sleep disorders and type 2 diabetes, where sleep disorders increase the risk of developing diabetes and vice versa, creating a vicious cycle (Sarkar et al., 2018).

There are various reasons in our modern world why we don't sleep well or don't have enough sleep. As we're social animals, we stay up very late, socialising with friends or work colleagues, or find our eyes glued to the screen and cannot leave our devices alone, whether for work or fun. These practices which we have normalised, can lead to diabetes. On the other hand, diabetes can cause sleep disorders, as we wake during the night to make repeated trips to the bathroom, to have a drink due to thirst, or because of a headache. All these are symptoms of unstable glucose levels. Obstructive sleep apnoea is also a common feature of diabetics. This is a sleep disorder where the individual's breathing is repeatedly interrupted as they sleep and has characteristic loud snoring with episodes of nonbreathing. I recommend you discuss this with your doctor if you or someone close to you has observed this pattern.

Importance of sleep: A good night's sleep should be peaceful, restful, and relaxing. Good quality sleep is important for health and general wellness. We're less likely to get ill, and it can help us lose weight. Sleep affects the brain in several ways. It restores the body and mind, stores memories, and can improve focus and performance. It can also remove toxins that build up during our waking hours. Lack of sleep is the direct opposite. The sleep experts suggest that we need an average of seven to nine hours of sleep daily. This may vary in individuals.

Here is a summary of the benefits of a good night's sleep in restoring the body and mind:

Tissue repair: During sleep, our body produces and releases hormones that promote tissue repair and growth, helping to repair damaged tissues, heal injuries, and build muscle.

Memory consolidation: Sleep plays an important role in our memory consolidation, helping us solidify new information and integrate it into existing knowledge and experience.

Our immune system function: Sleep helps to regulate our immune system and boosts its ability to fight off infections and illnesses.

Hormone regulation: Sleep helps to regulate our hormonal levels, including those that control appetite, metabolism, and stress response.

Energy restoration: Sleep provides a chance for the body to recharge its energy stores, helping to ensure that you wake up feeling refreshed and ready to tackle the day.

Story: Daren, a 41-year-old male attended a review in the diabetic clinic. Daren works from home. His HbA1c had risen to 78mmol/mol from 63mmol/mol in 6 months. On discussion, he explained that his diet was good. He had attended the diabetic educational class and was keeping to a low carb, low sugar diet. He had eliminated all processed food and had started going to the gym. When asked why he thought his HbA1c has gone up, he sadly explained that it was his flatmates. Daren has sleep apnoea. He was referred to the sleep clinic and was given a sleep device called CPAP, continuous positive airway pressure (CPAP) to help with his snoring and breathing. Unfortunately, this hasn't worked. Sometimes, his flatmates will knock on his door and call out that his snoring was keeping them awake. Other times, they would complain in the morning that they were unable to sleep due to his noisy sleeping habits. As a result, he's now reluctant to go to bed at night. He tries to sleep during the day when everyone is away, as he's scared to fall asleep at night. This has made him anxious and withdrawn. He feels that his flatmates are upset with him, and he tries to avoid them. This shows how stress can affect your blood glucose readings.

Walking

Walking is one of the recommended exercises for type 2 diabetics as well as for the entire human race. It's a great place to start when you think of increasing your physical activity. There's always a health benefit when you're moving as opposed to being sedentary. Adapting a walking habit bestows additional health benefits. Where you are physically doesn't matter; it's where you are mentally. You can create happiness through walking. Williams and Penman describe happiness as *"looking at the same things with different eyes."* They talk about how to find peace in a frantic world.

Most of us will consider walking a necessary act or even a chore when a drive in a vehicle is impractical. We have to stand up and take our whole being from one destination to another. Mindful walking is being aware of this activity. We can walk to pick up a newspaper from the news agents or walk our dog, mindful when we combine it with appreciation for being present here and now. I discuss more on mindful walking in the next chapter.

We spend a lot of time today sitting down, working on our computers, watching television, and, more recently, engaging in Zoom and Teams meetings online. There's a greater risk of making our lives sedentary, as a lot of us adapt to working remotely triggered by the COVID pandemic. This sedentary behaviour has not always been the case, and it's not what humans have evolved to do. The absence of physicality can cause loss of muscle mass, increase obesity rates, increase risk of heart disease, and poor mental health. Brisk walking can help build stamina, burn excess calories, help us breathe better, and improve the heart function.

Some people may go for a walk if they feel stuck in important decisions they must make. Walking is a head clearer. Walking in the open air gives the mind time to listen to your thoughts or those of others and helps to find solutions you had never thought about.

Some clear advantages of walking are:

- Can be done anytime, anywhere and comes with no charge.
- Is easy on the joints. It strengthens the bones and muscles.
- Improves blood circulation to the legs.
- Helps digest of food.
- May promote weight loss.
- Can help the body use insulin more effectively.
- Can help reduce stress levels, anxiety, and depression symptoms.
- Helps clarity of thought and decision making.
- Can also help improve sleep.

How do we start walking?

The key is planning. Write down your plan so that it's not only in your mind but you can also see it. This way, you believe it's doable. Set goals that are specific and achievable. Set aside a certain amount of time during the day to walk, be it morning, your lunch break, or in the evening so that it becomes part of your routine. You can keep a journal of your walks, how you feel after your walks: clear thinking, energised, healthier, weight loss, happier, and more. Review and see how you've done at the end of the week. Don't be judgemental if your day doesn't go as planned and you don't achieve your goal on the day. Remember, having the right mindset is knowing that if you have a setback, you can get right back up and start again.

If walking outside is more of a challenge for some, you can start in your home/office by walking on the spot, while reading your emails, cooking in the kitchen, or even watching television or listening to content on your smart device.

In diabetes, diet is of great consideration, whether you're on oral medication or insulin, when you decide to start walking. Consider having a pre or post snack depending on when you last had a meal, think of how far you want to walk and your pace. Consider taking a snack along with you if you'll be walking more than an hour so that you can have it if needed during your walk. Have a diabetic ID and inform someone of your planned walk. There's more information on preparing for walks on diabetic websites like the Diabetes UK site, which gives you confidence to go walking even on your own.

You might want to take this further and join a local walking group that meet regularly once a week or month. This is great for motivation and community spirit. You can also download smartphone apps like Mapmywalk or

Mapometer online which shows you walking routes in your area.

Story: Phil was 43 years old when he sent his diabetes into remission. His story was that he got motivated after accepting his diagnosis of type 2 diabetes, and he changed one thing. He attended the diabetic education class and simply started walking. When Phil was younger, he used to go to the gym regularly but stopped due to work pressures of running his company, and he failed to prioritise his health: exercise and diet. He thought about how he could incorporate both work and health to find a balance. Phil decided to choose an exercise that was realistic, and he could fit into his day. He chose walking.

Foot care

One of the risks of diabetes is foot complications or diabetic neuropathy, which can lead to amputations. It's important that we check and look after our feet to avoid this. Check your feet every day and look out for any changes. Checking after a walk is particularly important to notice any cuts, blisters, or callouses. Feel for pain and sensitivity in every area. Your health professional or team is the best advice source if you have any foot issues before embarking on heavy walking. Consider podiatry input at least once a year.

Simple footcare tips:

Quit smoking to improve blood circulation.

Check your feet every day and always wear socks with your footwear for your walk.

Nail clipping - be careful when cutting your nails to prevent cutting the skin by mistake as it can lead to other injuries that might be difficult to heal. Cut often but avoid cutting the nails too low and down the sides. Use nail clippers and emery board to file the corners. Avoid using sharp points of scissors; instead, use a nail brush to clean them.

Wash daily to prevent infection using simple soap and warm water. Moisturise daily. Don't let your feet dry out; on the other hand, don't infuse cream in between your toes, as that will cause wetness that might lead to infection.

Always check for loss of sensation and ingrowing toenails. Consult a foot specialist or your healthcare team who can refer you.

Wear fitting footwear that's not too tight or too loose to prevent rubbing. Ill-fitting shoes can cause foot problems even if they feel comfortable. The right shoes and socks will keep your feet healthy while you walk. It's good to choose broad fitting shoes with deep and rounded areas around the toes that are flat or with low heels. Shoes with laces, straps, or buckles can help the feet from sliding around. If stuck as to the choice of shoes, a podiatrist can help you make the right shoe choices. Visit a podiatrist at least once a year for a foot check, and your healthcare team can access your feet to determine whether you're at a high, medium, or low risk of developing foot problems.

Mindful walking

Mindful walking is more than just moving and setting down each foot in turn. As mentioned previously, it's paying attention to the sensations of our body and being aware of our surroundings and taking it in with all our senses. Tsang and his fellow researchers (2008) found that combining mindfulness with walking has been shown to improve both psychological and physiological health. The physical benefits of this combination are also apparent and can set the stage for other forms of physical activities.

Mindful walking is a mindfulness-based stress reduction technique which science has found to give positive rewards to our mental and physical wellness. Mindful walking can be performed anywhere, whether in woodlands of natural beauty or traffic-charged areas, as long as you remain present in the moment.

Though mindful walking can be practiced anywhere, when practiced in nature, the physical and mental gain are far reaching. We align ourselves with the world. We notice the trees, plants, flowers. We are one with them. As we breathe in oxygen and out carbon dioxide, there's a transfer process. We give them what they want, and they give us what we want, as they absorb carbon dioxide, and we inhale oxygen, which they release. What a symbiotic process!

We can walk mindfully by observing the sensations of the body. Noticing how the feet feel, the movement of the muscles and your steps as you walk, your balance and the way your arms swing. Having an open mind and being aware of your surroundings, enjoying and taking in the sights, sounds, and smells without judgement. This is all free, all you need is somewhere to walk, be it morning, afternoon, evening, or night or even during your lunch break at work. It's a simple practice we can all do, so long as we're able to walk and make the effort to fit this into your daily routine.

Don't let mobility issues stop you. You can still engage in cardiovascular, strength training and flexibility exercises.

Expect a backward move. It will happen. Don't be discouraged if you skip a few days or even a few weeks. Just get right back up and start again to slowly build up to your momentum. It becomes easier as your practice increases. This is life.

TIP: When walking put a smile on your face and be in the here and now. Be present.

Mindful eating

Remember, a mindful state develops over time and with regular daily practice, both formally and informally. Mindful eating is one form of behaviour modification that may help with weight loss. It's a practice that gives us the opportunity to appreciate food more and connect better with food, helping us make better food choices. This may in turn intervene with binge eating or emotional eating.

A mindful eater pays full attention to their food as they buy, prepare, serve, and consume it. We, however, should have the right mindset to adopt this practice, as it involves adjustments in the way we approach meals and snacks. Mindful eating can transform the way we think about food. If mindfulness means being present, then mindful eating points to being fully present while eating.

In this busy world, we often find ourselves multitasking with food. Some of us might start the morning horridly, grabbing a cup of coffee and pastry on the go, eating as they commute to work, have a working lunch break, and, on getting home, relax in front of the television for dinner. This might not necessarily be the case now, for many of us work from home. However, many times, we might have eaten something in the past couple of hours without paying much attention to the food and hardly tasting what we've eaten. In many instances, we struggle to remember what foods we've eaten in the day. Mindful eating is to practice avoiding internal distractions of our worries and thoughts and external distractions like smart devices and screens.

The Oxford University study found that the average UK male has increased in weight over 15 years between 1986 to 2000 by an average of 7.7kg. According to a 2011 report from the U.S. Department of Agriculture, the average American spends approximately two and a half hours per day consuming food while simultaneously engaged in other activities. These "busy" activities may include watching TV, working at a desk, or using a mobile device (U.S. Department of Agriculture, 2011).

As already mentioned, when we're working, driving, reading, watching television, or fiddling with a smart device, we're hardly aware of what we're eating. The lack of awareness, the mindless eating of what we ingest, could be contributing to the obesity epidemic and other associated health issues. Do you find that you tend to consume larger quantities of food when using electronic devices or scrolling through your phone, as opposed to intentionally sitting down at a table with family and friends? Research suggests that mindful eating practices, such as engaging in meaningful conversations about the food you are consuming, can promote more balanced eating habits (Zhu et al., 2020).

A few might think mindful eating is just trying to eat slowly and chewing food for a long time before swallowing. This is a good mindfulness exercise that makes you more relaxed and enjoy the eating experience, but there's more to mindful eating; it's about being aware of our thoughts, feelings, emotions, and physical perceptions associated with eating, it takes us back to our inborn wisdom about hunger and satiety.

Mindful eating allows us notice that we can make a positive choice with selecting and preparing food by listening to our inner wisdom, using all our senses to choose meals that will both satisfy and nourish our bodies.

Remember, mindfulness is always observing without judging. We acknowledge how we respond to food: do we like it, dislike it, or don't mind it? Are we aware of physical hunger and fullness, a signal for when to start eating or when to stop? This practice can help to reduce behaviours that are unhealthy such as emotional eating and overindulging in eating.

Qualities of a mindful eater

Accepts that there's no right or wrong way to eat; everyone can have their different degrees of awareness surrounding the experience of food.

Is aware of how they can make choices that support health and well-being.

Perceives the interconnection of earth, living beings, and cultural practices, and how food choices affect these systems.

Ways to practice a mindful eating exercise.

You can experiment with mindful eating by practicing with the "Mindful Eating Exercise." Before you eat anything, think of how this food or choice will help you, allowing yourself to become aware of the positive and nurturing opportunities that are available through food selection and preparation by respecting your own inner wisdom.

To implement a more structured approach to mindful eating, plan your meal before mealtimes. Write down two positive effects of your food choice. Keep a food journal. You can plan your meals a few days or a week ahead. You can, from time to time, assess your diet by turning back the pages to observe the many ways you're nurturing your body.

Here are some more tips.

Try to eat slowly, fully chew your food, savour, and enjoy the experience.

Notice and observe the different sensations while you eat, how it tastes, smells, feels, the colours, and the sound as you chew throughout the meal. Incorporating water as part of your meal can be a healthy way to stay hydrated and promote a feeling of fullness. One way to do this is to start your meal with a glass of water to help you feel full and prevent overeating.

Listen to your body and act, don't starve yourself, eat at mealtimes when you're hungry and stop when you begin to feel full, not continuing until uncomfortable because you're enjoying it or want to empty your plate.

Prepare or create dedicated times and space to eat, not on the go, not on your work desk, not watching television or on your phone, to enable you to focus on the food in front of you and avoid distractions. Eat on a real table when you can.

Enjoy the company of others, as these are moments of bonding and sharing the eating experience. Soft relaxing music may contribute to an enjoyable meal. Notice how every food can contribute towards a balanced diet, without judgement and guilt. Be compassionate towards yourself.

Regardless of whether you have disordered eating habits, wish to control your glucose levels, or want to lose weight, eating mindfully is something we can all benefit from.

You can see that the purpose of mindful eating isn't to lose weight, although there would most likely be weight loss if mindfully practiced; it's rather to help people to stop, be present, make better food choices, savour the moment, and enjoy the whole eating experience. The focus is on the experience, appreciation of food but not concerned about restricting intake. You choose what and how much you consume. However, it's no coincidence that by using a mindful approach, the choices are to eat less, savour more, and choose foods that will give the desired health benefits.

Some review studies have found a positive relationship between mindfulness-based interventions and weight loss when focused on reduction of food cravings and portion control. An article by Barnard et al. (2017), published in *ADA Diabetes Spectrum*, included mindfulness and mindful eating as part of a component of diabetes self-management education, along with other behaviour change programmes. It also showed positive results although inconclusive due to the way the study was carried out, as it was not clear whether it was mindful eating or other factors including exercise or sleep that contributed to a reduction in weight. The number of health professionals who believe that mindful eating can help people with diabetes to make a positive impact on their glucose levels by changing their eating pattern is increasing.

Olson and Emery in 2015 reviewed 19 studies that used a mindful eating approach. They found significant weight loss in 13 out of the 19 studies but they could not document the relationship between mindfulness and the observed weight loss. This is an indication that research is needed to better understand how mindfulness contributes to weight loss because there are limitations in the methods and differences between studies that affect the strength of the evidence. It's important to investigate how the mind, actions, and body are related to this, indicating that more research is needed to find this correlation, even though it's highly likely. Hence, they stated that the long-term effect of mindful eating in diabetes is unknown. The above earlier reviews did not focus on mindful eating as the primary outcome, as other factors like exercise and sleep were being considered. However, the review by Carolyn Dunn and colleagues in 2018, shows strong support for inclusion of mindful eating as a component for weight loss programs in treatment of overweight and obesity.

Don't skip this exercise. Try the "raisin experience" on eating mindfully. It's an exaggerated account that has become so popular due to the unevenness of a raisin.

Start by finding a quiet and comfortable place where you won't be disturbed for the next few minutes. Take a deep breath in, and exhale slowly, letting go of any tension in your body.

Now, find a raisin or imagine that you're holding a single raisin in your hand. Take a moment to examine it closely, really seeing it as if for the first time. Notice its size, shape, and colour, and the texture of the wrinkles on its surface.

Next, bring the raisin up to your nose and inhale deeply. Notice any aromas or scents that you can detect. Then, place the raisin on your tongue, but don't chew it yet. Just let it rest there for a moment and notice how it feels against your tongue and the roof of your mouth.

When you're ready, slowly begin to chew the raisin, but pay close attention to the entire experience. Notice the changing texture of the raisin as you chew it, and the way its flavour develops and changes over time. Take your time with each chew, really savouring the experience.

Finally, when you've finished chewing the raisin, swallow it, and notice how it feels as it goes down your throat. Take a moment to appreciate the entire experience, from beginning to end.

When you're ready, take another deep breath in, and exhale slowly. Bring your attention back to the present moment, feeling grounded and centred.

How was that for you?

The health benefits of mindful eating are stress reduction, improved digestion, reduced overeating, and decreased weight gain. Taking time to appreciate the small things we often miss can liberate us from our deep thoughts on our daily concerns.

Mindful eating helps individuals cultivate awareness of both internal and external triggers to eating, interrupts automatic eating, and promotes eating in response to the natural physiological cues of hunger and satiety. Mindful eating interventions have been effective in facilitating improvement in dysregulated eating and dietary patterns. Through practice over time, eating mindfully can interrupt habitual eating behaviours and provide greater regulation of food choice. More research is needed to determine the long-term impact of mindful eating programs.

Chapter 5: Breathing

"Feelings come and go like clouds in a windy sky. Conscious breathing is my anchor." —Thich Nhat Hanh

Did You Know?

We take about 1,000 breaths each hour, up to 25,000 breaths each day and probably an average of 100 million breaths over a lifetime.

Breathing is the process of moving air in and out the lungs to help with gas exchange in our bodies. We essentially breathe in oxygen and breathe out carbon dioxide. It's something we never think about. We just do it naturally. It's responsible for our lives. As humans, we can survive without food for weeks, without water for days, but without breathing for just a few minutes (approx. 1-4 minutes). Breathing is the only part of our autonomic nervous system that's both conscious and unconscious. Unconscious breathing has been this way for most of us. Breathing is often a reflection of how we feel. Breathing also changes how we feel. Breathing changes in response to different stimuli, noticed in reaction to a fight or flight response, in anger, anticipation, nervousness, happiness, bliss, etc. Notice how your breathing changes. The fight or flight response prepares our body for action. This reaction was extremely useful years ago when our ancestors lived in caves alongside wild animals. The reaction prepared them for running or fighting. We still possess these survival instincts and it can be useful when we need to act quickly, for example, escaping fire or avoiding a speeding vehicle. When this same fight or flight reaction is triggered by worrying thoughts about our health or imagining the worst from family or friends, it can have a detrimental effect on our physical and psychological well-being. The fight or flight response won't be useful in such circumstances and will make us feel worse. We release stress hormones, such as adrenaline and cortisol, that makes our blood sugar levels rise. This anxiety becomes a problem when it affects our everyday life and stops us from doing things that we need to do or wish to do.

When anxiety creeps in from the fight or flight reaction, adrenaline is released into the blood stream, setting up the body for action. This causes a number of physical changes such as:

(a) Head: sweating, blushing, blurred vision, and dry mouth.

(b) Breathing: shallow and rapid breath, palpitations, chest pain, tingling, feelings of faintness or dizziness, and aching muscles.

(c) Abdominal/excretory: churning sensation, nausea, indigestion, urinary urgency, and diarrhoea.

These unpleasant feelings aren't harmful in the short term but can lead to more severe problems if the anxiety or stressful situation becomes repeated or prolonged. As these hormones are released, they can cause the liver to release stored glucose into the bloodstream for energy. This can lead to a rapid increase in blood sugar levels, which is problematic for individual with diabetes who have difficulty regulating their sugar levels. In the long term, repeated episodes of elevated sugar levels due to the fight or flight response can contribute to the development of diabetic complications such as nerve damage, kidney disease, and cardiovascular disease. We need to recognise the fight or flight situations and act accordingly to manage these symptoms to be more in control and to prevent it from building up. We will regularly encounter anxiety or stress in our lives, but how we deal with it makes all the difference.

Conscious breathing

In this chapter, I explore how conscious breathing can have positive effects on us. Conscious breathing is when we breathe with awareness, intention, and attention to our inner experience and in the present moment. It's the way we breathe in oxygen, which oxygenates our body in a more efficient manner, and realising its benefits on our thoughts, emotions, and body functions.

This is also known as breathwork. Hendricks and Brown (2021) have described breathwork as various techniques and practices that involve controlled breathing patterns for the purpose of improving physical, mental, and emotional well-being. It's a therapeutic approach that utilizes the breath as a tool for accessing and releasing emotions, reducing stress, and promoting relaxation. Breathwork has been shown to have a positive impact on managing type 2 diabetes by reducing stress, improving blood sugar control, and increasing insulin sensitivity. One example of a breathing exercise that may be helpful for diabetics is the "4-7-8" breath, which involves inhaling for a count of 4, holding the breath for a count of 7, and exhaling for a count of 8. Practicing this technique for several minutes each day may help to lower blood sugar levels and improve overall well-being. I would always recommend you consult with a healthcare professional before starting any new exercise or breathing program.

Here's a simple demonstration that can be used universally for relaxed breathing, which I've put together based on various practices I've encountered. Let's practice!

This breathing exercise can be done anywhere, your home, workplace, before a presentation or a speech, etc. It gets you to calmness to embrace your inner self. You can play soft music in the background if you want.

1. Get into a nice comfortable position. Place your hands on both sides of your upper stomach, just under your ribs.

2. Count from 1 to 4 as you gently and steadily breathe in through your nose, feeling your stomach rise, pushing against your hands.

3. Count from 1 to 8 as you slowly and evenly breathe out through your mouth as if you're blowing air into a straw, feeling your stomach sinking. As you breathe out, say a word or phrase which helps you relax. For example, 'I am calm' or 'I am relaxed'.

Do this three times.

4. Begin to breathe at a natural pace for yourself. Notice the way your stomach rises when you breathe in and goes back when you breathe out.

Now you've got the breathing rhythm.

5. As you breathe in slowly, close your eyes tightly then let your eyes relax as you breathe out (repeat x3).

6. Move over to your mouth. Breathe in holding your mouth tightly and clenching your teeth, breathe out and relax your mouth and jaws, your mouth feeling soft and comfortable (repeat x3).

7. Shoulders. Breathe in and raise your shoulders up and back, breathe out and lower your shoulders slowly to a relaxing position (repeat x3)

8. Arms. Breathe in as you stretch both arms straight out in front of you and make a fist with your hands. Breathe out and release your clenched fist then slowly bring them down (repeat x3). Relax your arms and the shoulders and feel the difference.

9. Legs. Hold your legs out in front of you. Point your toes forward, wiggle them. Breathe in, then out and slowly let them relax (repeat x3)

Keep breathing in deeply through your nose and out slowly through your mouth and feel how relaxed and calm your whole body feels.

Now return to breathing normally. **How was that for you?**

This simple relaxed breathing exercise can be easily adapted, as it works fast, lowers stress, and can be done anywhere.

We all have control over the way we breathe because it's always with us; it's part of our being. Most of us breathe incorrectly. We shallow breathe using our intercostal muscles and inhale minimal air into our lungs instead of breathing deeply from our diaphragm. Shallow breathing is usually more rapid can lead to hyperventilation. It disrupts the oxygen carbon dioxide balance. The longer inhalation and exhalation slow the heart rate and improves blood pressure. A decrease in blood pressure can result in a reduction in cortisol, which is a stress hormone that accelerates ageing.

Taking control of the way we choose to breathe is a step in the right direction. Conscious breathing practice can vary in duration, intensity, and purpose. In addition to relaxation, it can help us focus, boost energy, and relieve stress and trauma. When practiced regularly, it becomes a habit you can use whenever the situation calls for it. It's a training to breathe well.

Conscious breathing isn't yoga, meditation, or mindfulness. It forms the basis for any practice as in psychological therapies, yoga, and meditation and in many sports or physical exercises in preparation and cooling down phases. It's not limited to any age and could be learnt in workplaces, schools, or at home.

Diaphragmatic breathing (belly breathing) is a conscious breathing exercise that involves the diaphragm, stomach, and abdominal muscles. It helps a person use their diaphragm to support their breath. The diaphragm is a sheet of large muscle that separates the thoracic cavity, where the heart and lungs lie from the abdominal cavity. It plays an important part in respiration. It helps to move air in and out of the lungs. When you breathe in air through your nose, the diaphragm contracts downwards, the volume of the thoracic cavity increases as air is being drawn into the lungs. It's best to start this breathing exercise while lying down comfortably, and when you get used to this practice, you can be seated or standing. Belly breathing ensures you get enough oxygen into the lungs for distribution. This form of breathing controls complications attributed to high sugar levels.

Breathing right: This is the process of taking in enough air through your nostrils, to enable optimal oxygenation and exhaling the right amount of carbon dioxide to find the right balance for effective functioning of the body's internal processes.

Breathing right can help cure or control diabetes through weight loss. When we breathe wrong or our breath is shallow, it triggers the fight or flight sympathetic response, causing the production of cortisol, the stress hormone. The body starts storing energy in the form of glucose for the impending attack as primal instincts take over. This can cause the liver to release more glucose into the bloodstream. This increase in blood glucose provides energy for the body to respond to the perceived threat. However, if the body does not use up all the extra glucose, it can accumulate in the brain and contribute to elevated blood sugar levels which can lead to changes in the balance of hormones and chemicals in the brain, that can make you feel hungry and increase glucose demand. When you eat sugary or starchy foods, it can make the problem worse and keep the cycle going. A lot of people gain weight because they're not breathing right. Improper breathing patterns may contribute to unhealthy eating habits and decreased physical activity levels, which can lead to weight gain. When we breathe shallowly, our bodies may not receive sufficient oxygen, which can lead to feelings of fatigue and stress. This can result in a lack of motivation to engage in physical activity, leading to a sedentary lifestyle. Shallow breathing can also lead to a build-up of carbon dioxide in the body, which can trigger feelings of anxiety and stress, and can lead to emotional eating. On the other hand, breathing right can help us lose weight as the fight or flight response isn't activated. It enables us manage stress better, reduce feelings of anxiety, and increase overall energy levels. Breathing in enough oxygen helps in optimal gas exchange and promotes our overall wellness.

A person with a good breathing pattern will take about 2 hours to digest a regular meal whereas a wrong breather will take more than twice the time to process the same food.

Breathwork can be a valuable addition to your overall wellness routine. There is a wealth of resources online to help you explore different breathing techniques such as slow breathing and nasal breathing. By utilizing these practices, you can experience their numerous benefits. Fortunately, there are a variety of apps and online resources that you can access through your phone or computer, making it convenient to learn and practice from anywhere. With so much information available, there's certainly a lot to discover and explore. You'll be amazed at the difference breathing consciously will make in your day-to-day living. It is, however, important to consult your healthcare professional before you engage in activities you are unsure of.

Mindful breathing

Breathing mindfully is different from a mindful breathing exercise or conscious breathing. You're not trying to perfect your breathing, rather you're an observer. Mindful breathing helps to focus on the present moment. It has a positive impact on both physical and mental health. By focusing on your breath and staying present in the moment, you can alleviate worries about past regrets or the unpredictable future and reduce negative thinking, anxiety, and stress.

Mindful breathing can also be helpful for managing burnout and certain types of chronic pain. It's a simple and you can incorporate into your daily routine.

Mindfulness can be practiced by everybody, and breathing mindfully is no exception. It's good practice to stop ourselves and pay attention or observe what our body does automatically. Observing your breathing without judgement is a great way of focusing the mind to be present.

Mindful breathing involves being in a relaxed position, seated or lying, so that you're breathing freely without constriction.

You can do this yourself quietly or with calming music in the background or you can play a guided meditation recording. If you're conscious of time, you can set a timer; otherwise, you can meditate as long as you want. There are many guided meditation videos you can access from the internet, or you can download an app onto your smartphone.

Notice your breathing as you breathe in and out. How does it feel to inhale? Is it deep or shallow, long or short, catchy or smooth? What about the space at the end of the inhale before you begin to exhale? How is your exhale and the space before you inhale again. Notice if your inhale breath is cooler than your exhale breath or if it's not. Just observe, no judgement.

Observe your body as you focus on how you feel when you breathe. Where do you feel your breath most? How does breathing through your nostrils feel? Are both nostrils clear? Or does one feel easier to breathe through than the other? Are your inhales felt more in the chest, shoulders, or deep down in your belly?

It's fine for your mind to wander; acknowledge this without judgement and bring it back to your breath and observations of your breathing body.

Once your allocated time is up, notice how you feel. Notice how your body feels. Are you more relaxed? Remember there's no right or wrong way. Sometimes, it can take time to breathe mindfully, as you find yourself losing focus and not being present. Don't be discouraged; keep practicing, and, once hacked, you'll see the benefits.

According to Judson Brewer, staying curious and being aware of your breath rather than trying to perfect your breathing always will help you focus and create less worry about right or wrong breathing.

Yoga

Yoga is an ancient practice originating in India. It's a practice of physical, mental, and spiritual disciplines. Yoga, in modern terms and especially in the Western world, signifies a posture-based physical fitness, stress-relief, and/or relaxation techniques like breathing. The word "yoga" means "to unite." The aim is to unite body, mind, and spirit as well as the individual self and universal consciousness. A body of evidence suggests that people with diabetes can benefit from yoga practices. Practising yoga is likely to help with glycaemic control and can lower oxidative stress in type 2 diabetes. Yoga also has a positive effect in reduction of high blood pressure, improving mood, and promoting good sleep. Everyone can practice yoga. Yoga breathing should be slow, full, and deep, breathing in through your nose and out through your nose. There are so many yogic breathing exercises out there. Yoga breathing exercise is also known as pranayama which is a Sanskrit word meaning "breath control." It's a collection of different breathing techniques that the ancient yogis used for healing, purification, and rejuvenating mental focus. "Prana" means "life force energy, breath of life, energy" and "Yama" means "control, constraint." This is the main component in the practice of yoga. Amazing things can happen when you control your breath and regulate the flow of life force within the body. Andrew Weil endorses yoga by saying, "Practicing a regular, mindful breathing exercise can be calming and energizing and can even help with stress-related health problems ranging from panic attacks to digestive disorders." My advice will be to try different yoga exercises to see which ones resonate with you. Many people are put off because their first experience with yoga wasn't what they expected. There's the yogic breathing in conjunction with the exercise. Below are some of the best yoga breathing exercises as described in the Awaken.com website at https://awaken.com/2021/02/the-10-best-yoga-breathing-exercises/. Some expertise might be required to practice some of them and should be practiced under the guidance of a qualified yoga teacher, especially if you're new to pranayama. Consult with your healthcare practitioner for suitability.

Why don't you pause from reading and see which ones you might be interested in?

Below are brief summaries of the 10 breathing techniques discussed in the article:

Nadi Shodhana (Alternate Nostril Breathing): This technique involves breathing through alternate nostrils and can help balance the left and right hemispheres of the brain, as well as calm the mind and reduce stress.

Kapalabhati (Breath of Fire): This technique involves quick, forceful exhales followed by passive inhales, and can help improve respiratory function, increase energy, and clear the mind.

Ujjayi (Ocean Breath): This technique involves inhaling and exhaling through the nose while constricting the back of the throat, creating an ocean-like sound, and can help calm the mind and increase focus.

Bhastrika (Bellows Breath): This technique involves rapid, forceful inhales and exhales, and can help improve lung capacity, increase energy, and improve mental clarity.

Sitali (Cooling Breath): This technique involves inhaling through a curled tongue or pursed lips and can help cool the body and calm the mind.

Sitkari (Hissing Breath): This technique involves inhaling through the teeth while keeping the lips closed and can help reduce stress and cool the body.

Bhramari (Bee Breath): This technique involves making a humming sound while exhaling, and can help reduce stress, calm the mind, and improve concentration.

Murcha (Swooning Breath): This technique involves inhaling deeply and holding the breath and can help improve focus and increase energy.

Plavini (Floating Breath): This technique involves swallowing air and holding it in the stomach and can help improve digestion and reduce bloating.

Sama Vritti (Equal Breathing): This technique involves inhaling and exhaling for an equal amount of time and can help balance the nervous system and improve focus.

How did you find them?

Oxygen transported into the body through inhalation, kickstarts energy production for various processes in the body. We breathe unconsciously every time. Imagine what happens when you do it consciously.

Story: Kofi, 43-year-old male had been living with type 2 diabetes for 4 years. Despite taking his medication and watching his diet, he found that his blood sugar levels were still often too high. He felt frustrated and helpless, until one day, he read about the benefits of breathing exercises for managing diabetes.

John decided to give it a try and began incorporating a simple breathing exercise, known as the "4-7-8" breath, into his daily routine. He inhaled for a count of four, held his breath for a count of seven, and exhaled for a count of eight. He practiced this technique for several minutes each day.

To his surprise, after a few weeks, John's blood sugar levels began to stabilize. He felt more relaxed and in control of his diabetes. He also started incorporating mindfulness and meditation into his daily routine, which helped him to manage his stress levels.

John continued to practice his breathing exercises and mindfulness techniques and soon was able to reduce his diabetes medication. He felt healthier and more energized than he had in years.

From that day on, John made sure to make time for his breathing exercises and mindfulness practices every day. He was grateful for the positive impact it had on his diabetes and on his overall well-being. He also recommended it to his friends and family who were living with diabetes, and they too experienced positive results.

I have taken you out of the traditional practice of diabetes care of using medication, diet, and physical activity, and have focused more on breathing exercises, in this chapter especially. This is because breathing exercises that involve slowing down the breath have become increasingly popular in the Western world, as they are believed to have various health benefits. However, despite their growing popularity, these practices are not widely embraced by the medical community as we await more research to be done to investigate their potential health benefits and to determine how they can be used most effectively. In the meantime, individuals who practice slow breathing techniques often report feeling more relaxed, less anxious, and better able to manage stress. This is an encouragement to practice various techniques and see which ones resonates with you.

Chapter 6: Journaling

"Journal writing gives us insights into who we are, who we were, and who we can become" —Sandra Marinella

Journaling is for everyone, both young and old. Many of us kept diaries in our younger years, but as time went on, we completely abandoned this important practice. As adults, keeping a journal effectively can impact our lives positively in various ways. The act of journaling isn't just a good and mindful practice, its benefits are far reaching.

How we derive benefit

Writing can be therapeutic, providing a way to process and make sense of difficult experiences, and to gain insight and perspective on one's life. It can be used to improve overall physical health and mental wellbeing particularly when trying to monitor or keep blood glucose levels stable. Increased memory and creativity are also benefits of journaling.

There's no specific way to journal. It certainly can look different for everyone. Some people may prefer to use a notebook or electronic device (phone or computer). You may carry a notebook with you always to jot down notes as you go along your daily activities, to capture ideas, for reminders, experiences, or events as they happen, or you might journal at the end of the day or even first thing in the morning. Your journaling might be a few lines of bullet points on a page or comprehensive writing, covering pages. Whichever is your style, all that's important is writing down information about yourself, your thoughts, and your day, to allow you gain insight on how you're doing. You'll realise this when you write it down on paper or type into your device. The good thing about journaling is that you can look back and compare various days, see what's working, what hasn't worked or what you could do better. It creates better thinking habits. When you begin to communicate with yourself on paper, you'll become better at describing what you want to say to others, and they understand you better. Your confidence increases and your communication increases.

You may want to own a gratitude journal, a food and activity journal or even a future-self journal. Journaling makes you more self-aware. You become connected to yourself. It can get you to become thankful for what you have now and become aware of your future goals. Some people have more than one journal for different purposes as they like to keep their thoughts and emotions separate from their daily activities. Start off with one journal and see what works for you.

Many people who have had diabetes for some time might already be keeping a food and activity journal which helps in blood glucose control. A few of my patients have described how journaling gets them to think and plan. It can help you understand obstacles and realise your strengths. You'll be able to sort out your thoughts, fears, and feelings, resolve problems, acknowledge successes, and rationalise information coming from all angles. When you look back in your journal, you might notice patterns such as blood glucose dipping or rising, developing headaches, getting indigestion or abdominal upset at particular times of the day, week or month which might be as a result of certain foods you eat and when you eat them. Journaling could be conversational. Conversing with yourself and recognising negative patterns will enable you to implement changes to better manage your blood glucose levels.

There are also other benefits of journaling that can't be measured but can ease the burdens of type 2 diabetes such as your fluctuating moods, stress, and depressive symptoms which can raise blood glucose levels. Journaling can make you recognise your own habits and question yourself. What's causing your overwhelm, increasing weight, poor eating habits, and feeling unwell? Through journaling, you may become aware of the source of the stress, have conversations with yourself, and arrive at solutions to create new and better behaviours.

When you write down your thoughts, emotions, feelings, and experiences, you can make choices and decisions about lifestyle: food, exercise, and medication. If you're accountable and true to yourself, you might choose not to have that extra slice and extra drink.

When you look over your setbacks and accomplishments, you might get inspired on moving forward. You may identify what's not serving you well and what you've done well. You can draw inspiration from the good then make some changes to soar even higher. You'll notice the progress over time.

The art around journaling

A journal is your own book. It's up to you to select your style, colour, and size. You might decide to choose pages that are lined or blank sheets. You can write in different pen colours to represent certain areas of your journaling or the same colour of pen or even put your thoughts down in sections, such as sections for your diet, exercise, thoughts, goals, and relationships. Others might be more artistic and want to draw. You can be flexible with your choice. A journal that serves you today might not be the right one for you tomorrow. Really take time to choose your journal, as what you write in it will be worth a million times more in health and wealth benefits than the cost of it. Putting things down on paper can transform your whole life. When you write you goals in your journal, a message is sent to your brain that says, “This is crucial to me.” This is your space where you can dream and make these dreams a reality.

You might have heard about “bullet journaling” developed by Ryder Carroll in 2013, carefully laid out and well thought of. It was said to be for the digital age and set out to maximise reflection, ideation, and dedication where your daily entry helps to declutter your mind by easily putting your ideas on paper, which you can go back to later. There are quite a few similar fancy journals that can be bought online or purchased in bookstores. My style however is simple. I have dated diaries or notebooks that I use to write things down and can write as much as I want, depending on how I feel on the day. The constant for me is being consistent and noting the dates of my entries.

In 2018, nearly 210 million dollars was spent on journaling supplies. However due to the pandemic when schools were studying remotely and a lot of companies were setting up virtually, back to school supplies and retail office work supplies went down in demand. This downturn hardly affected the demand for journals and notebooks; instead, it thrived as more people got in touch with their inner being through writing. An alternative option is using your phone or electronic device. As I was writing this part of the book, I decided to keep a digital daily journal using an app I downloaded onto my phone. I must admit that at the beginning, it didn't quite flow as well as writing on paper, and I missed a few days of journaling as I tried to form this new habit. It feels more natural to me now and this is a typical example of how difficult habits are to build, but, through persistence, you'll succeed. I have gone back to my traditional pen and paper writing but often use my app during the day when I'm out and about and need to note anything of importance.

Here is a summary of handwriting vs. electronic device: If you use both methods of journaling, handwriting and electronic devices, you're getting the best of both worlds. Handwriting stimulates memory retention and creativity, while electronic devices offer convenience and accessibility. It's important to strike a balance between the two, using handwriting when you want to focus on memory retention or unleash your creativity, and electronic devices when you want to quickly jot down notes or access information on-the-go. The potential drawbacks of each method are physical strain from handwriting for any reason and distraction from electronic devices. You can use either method appropriately or enjoy the benefits of both.

When you think about the benefits of journaling, what's a good trigger to remind you? Setting an alarm might help at first to form the habit of writing things down: a thought, an action, a plan, that achievement or disappointment, that win.

Toni Rodriguez, in 2013, wrote about the use of expressive writing to heal wounds. He explained the research that wounds can heal faster through writing expressively your thoughts and feelings The study was on 49 healthy adults between the ages of 64 to 97 who were instructed to write for 20 minutes, three consecutive days, either about upsetting events or their daily activities. A two-week delay was observed to ensure any negative emotions were no longer affecting the participants. Following this, all subjects underwent a biopsy on their arm, and the healing process was photographed over the next 21 days. On the 11th day, it was discovered that the group that did expressive writing had a 76 percent recovery rate, whereas the control group had a 42 percent recovery rate.

When an individual experiences long-term emotional distress, it can lead to an increase in the production of stress hormones, such as cortisol, which can ultimately weaken the immune system. However, it has been suggested that expressive writing may have a positive impact on the body's cortisol levels. By writing about emotional topics, participants may have been able to alleviate some of the stress and ultimately lower their cortisol levels.

In addition to the potential impact of expressive writing on cortisol levels, it's possible that the study's positive outcomes could also be attributed to the participants' improved sleep patterns. It was observed that those who had more sleep in the week leading up to the biopsy had a faster healing process, likely because sleep is known to play a critical role in various bodily processes associated with healing. Therefore, it's possible that the combined effect of both expressive writing and better sleep may have contributed to the participants' faster recovery times

The act of writing evokes mindfulness, reduces stress, can help to achieve goals, improves emotional intelligence, can reduce symptoms of depression, and improve memory. Journaling can help improve your sleep, increase productivity, and improve your physical health. The develop-good-habits website describes some benefits of journaling. For more detailed reading on journaling, go to https://www.developgoodhabits.com/benefits-journaling/.

Setting goals are important. According to Antoine de Saint-Exupery, "A goal without a plan is just a wish." Write down goals on how to go about achieving your ideal food plan, weight, mindfulness practice, or work/home commitments. Starting small with specific and challenging goals is the key. Introduce one new thing at a time. Don't try to change a lot at once. Remember, what we do helps us achieve goals, and we become what we repeatedly do.

Use your journal entries as a textbook for life or make your digital entry an eBook for life. Make time and go back to read your journals at least once a month, you'll see how far you've come.

A personal journal

Here is a journal by a friend who has found comfort in journaling:

I prefer writing on paper. I buy a different cover journal every time the last one gets filled. As I fill up my notebook, I really look forward to my next purchase.

I have just turned forty-three and I have been living with diabetes for 2 years. When I became aware I had type 2 diabetes, I was confused and in slight denial. I say slight because I knew about diabetes as my mum has type 2 diabetes, but I didn't think I would have it too. For the next two months, I conveniently ignored my new diagnosis and carried on as if this news was about someone else. Until one day, I said to myself, "Who do you think you are kidding? You better take control; otherwise, you will find yourself in the passenger's seat." I started studying and researching about diabetes. I became really interested and read a lot about having a positive attitude towards change, food, exercise, and emotional well-being. I came across how reflective writing could affect my thoughts, my food habits, and how physical activity could have a great impact on diabetic control. My HbA1c was 56mmol/mol (7.3%) at the time of diagnosis. I kept getting lots of headaches and passing urine frequently. It became an issue because my sleep was being affected from waking up two to three times at night. My doctor recommended a blood test, and the result came back with a high blood sugar level and HbA1c. I was told by my doctor that getting my HbA1c down to less than 48mmol/mol puts me in the range of a non-diabetic, however, still pre-diabetic, unless I go down to below 42mmol/mol. I was now familiar with the numbers, and I understood what she meant. From the onset, I divided my journal into sections. Every day, I will keep a food diary of what, when and how! What did I eat? When did I eat? and how did I feel when I ate? I was happy to invest in a blood glucose monitor and I checked my blood glucose reading twice a day for three days of the week just to give me an idea of how the food I eat causes a spike in my blood sugar levels. I became a woman with a mission. I wrote my first shopping list in my journal. I also added a treat, a bar of dark chocolate. At the bottom of my list, it read, "I am very proud of me at how healthy my food list looks." Since then, I write my weekly shopping list and I then I add one treat at the end to reward myself. I keep a daily journal about my activities. I noticed that walking contributed to keeping me in shape but also allowed me to ponder on my thoughts, ask questions about myself, my fears about diabetes, and my future. Writing things down in my journal made me feel like I had a companion, and I would almost always find my answers there, find comfort. Things become clearer whenever I journal. I appreciate everything around me. I notice the leaves on the trees, the butterflies, insects, birds, animals all living their own lives in this planet. Colours are more vibrant, smells, sounds of humans, the universe, more distinct. This is how journaling makes me feel. It alters my perception and I feel in tune with the universe.

Two years on, I've got my diabetes under control. At my last check, my HbA1c reading was 47mmol/mol. It fluctuates between 47 and 49mmol/mol. I had asked my doctor to give me the opportunity to try without medication and she has been very supportive. I did it! I have been told I only need a yearly check now. My next aim is to get it down to below 42mmol/mol and I am certain I can do it, as I have developed lasting habits that serve me.

For whoever is reading this, I urge you to take a pen and write on paper or use a device to take regular notes. Any how you want to do it. You can even record your thoughts. No formal writing is required, and you are not being graded. No one has to read this. It is just for you to be honest with yourself and the way you feel. You can express your anger and disappointment with the system, your friends or even family who are not supportive. You can also celebrate your wins, express gratitude for the support you have received, your victories in managing your diabetes, and further plans.

Journaling helps filter out overload of information you receive from the media which tends to be confusing and often makes you feel guilty that you are not following every suggestion from the "experts." I am my own expert. Journaling helps me focus on my own method as diabetes should be personalised to the individual. It wasn't easy at first. It still isn't. Sometimes, life gets in the way; I don't judge myself if I go on for days without writing. I know the benefits and feel better anytime I journal. It is now a worthwhile habit. Start writing, anything at first, gratitude journaling, mindful writing anything that comes to mind. It is the act of writing that counts. The more you write, the better you will feel. —Candy

In summary, journaling is a personal and creative process that can be tailored to meet the unique needs and preferences of each individual. It can be a powerful tool for self-reflection, personal growth, and emotional well-being. I have listed some advantages to recap:

1. Self-reflection: Journaling provides a space for individuals to reflect on their thoughts, feelings, and experiences, which can help them gain insight and perspective on their lives.
2. Stress reduction: Writing about difficult experiences or emotions can help to process and release them, which can lead to reduced stress and anxiety.
3. Goal setting: Journaling can help individuals to set and track goals, which can increase motivation and accountability.

4. Memory retention: Writing about events and experiences can help to solidify memories, making them more easily accessible in the future.
5. Problem solving: Writing about problems or challenges can help to clarify thoughts and emotions, which can make it easier to find solutions.
6. Creativity: Journaling can be a creative outlet, allowing individuals to experiment with different writing styles and forms of expression.
7. Emotional regulation: Journaling allows people to express and understand their emotions, which is an important aspect of emotional regulation.
8. Personal Growth: It can help individuals understand their patterns of behaviour and thoughts, which can aid in personal growth and self-improvement.
9. Medical Management: Journaling can be particularly useful for people living with chronic medical conditions, such as diabetes, as it allows them to track symptoms, medication, and progress over time.
10. Therapeutic: Journaling can be therapeutic, and it can be used as a form of self-care and self-help.

"Start writing, no matter what. The water does not flow until the faucet is turned on" —Louis L'Amour.

Turn on your faucet. Start writing and let it flow.

Chapter 7: Community

"The world is so empty if one thinks only of mountains, rivers and cities; but to know someone who thinks and feels with us, and who, though distant, is close to us in spirit, this makes the earth for us an inhabited garden." —Goethe

Do you feel alone with your condition and are still asking the questions or wondering how to do this on your own? Are you the kind of person who needs encouragement and support but feels that you'll also need something extra to keep you going, such as people with comparative conditions, in addition to your family's and friends' support? This isn't unusual, and it's highly encouraged, as it's easy to feel self-pity, sadness, and regret.

You might want to join a community with similar issues. There are many diabetic support groups around the globe. Some are more well-known than others. The larger groups are Diabetic UK and American Diabetic Association. If you would like to meet face to face, you can search online for local groups in your area. There are also several diabetes awareness programmes too.

Sense of belonging

There's no telling the advantage of being part of a community. First, it will make you realise that you're not alone. You'll pick up tips that will help you manage your diabetes better. Groups can be quite inspirational and motivational. People who might be doing amazing things can give you inspiration to be bolder or more aggressive to achieve your desired goals.

Learning and sharing

You'll discover new foods and plans, and you can share your own experience as well. At times, when you feel like your motivation is weaning, being in a group keeps you going. The right group will help you modify your lifestyle and make changes.

Not every group is the right fit for you. For example, if you have type 2 diabetes and you join a type 1 group, being there would be of little benefit to you. There are a few points to consider before deciding which group to join, be it online or face-to-face gatherings.

Openness and friendships

There should be an instant feeling of warmth that you're welcome to the group. You're free to express your fears without feeling ashamed or guilty and not being judged. Others are willing to share their lows and their success stories and give positive criticism and encouragement in a relaxed atmosphere. Most of these groups come with little or no financial tag.

In the UK, prediabetics are referred to diabetes prevention programmes to prevent them from onward development of diabetes. They're kept under the radar and recalled annually for blood tests and reviews. The educational programmes can sometimes become the initial setting to start forming relationships. The same also applies to newly diagnosed diabetics who are encouraged to attend a structured education programme that explains more about the diabetic journey. The feedback from patients is mostly positive. The great advantage of the programme is that you can reattend if needed after a couple of years as a refresher.

Some of us already belong to mastermind communities in our various works of life, where we align with people of like minds and gain a lot from one another, pushing us along to dare to do things we would not normally have imagined. Most new members are amazed at how bonds are instantly formed and compassion is shown among members.

Gone are the days when having diabetes was a kept secret. Life can be put at risk by not coming forward with symptoms you're experiencing or not going to a medical professional for help. Such situations cause a lot of emotional stress and worsen diabetes. There are a lot of diabetic awareness groups and care lines that can be accessed. Such places can be found simply by searching on the internet.

We need to realise that fear is the number one contributory factor to hiding diabetes from others. It could be fear of being discriminated or bullied at work and being made fun off by friends who don't understand this condition. Talking about diabetes is a great way to create awareness in people around you, and they, in turn, can spread the message.

The benefit of belonging to a community cannot be overemphasised, as it brings a sense of belonging. We cannot exist on our own. Human beings are social beings, even though opinions might differ. There's the possibility that in a diabetic community whose members are supportive and have similar values, a unified voice can give strength to change and influence proposals for new ways to manage diabetes and even affect legislation positively. There will be unending tips, ideas, and advice on how others have managed their diabetes through diet, exercise, or other lifestyle changes. Rather than learning from trials and errors, we could ask the community if someone has experienced the same issue we're facing, which could be useful to our situation. We can explore suggestions and adapt to suit our own lifestyle.

We can develop contacts. People tend to align with certain individuals in the community who might have strong contacts and who can introduce them to places they want to go or people they want to meet. They get the opportunity to involve themselves in interesting activities through the people they meet; they can have meetups and engage in other social activities that can be for fun or for business opportunities, which adds to our overall life experience.

Story: Forty-nine-year-old Lara had an unfavourable experience in a virtual diabetes community that she joined. She had confessed to the group about her struggles of not being able to give up desserts after lunch. She had a thing for cheesecakes and had been having half her usual portion for the past week and was unable to completely stop. She was expecting understanding and empathy but was hurt by one of the replies that was directed at her bluntly: "If you're determined, you have no excuse not to stop!" She explained that what really upset her was that nobody in the group reprimanded the attacker, even though there were others in the group who were encouraging with a mild statement of "be nice." Lara came off the group and decided not to join any other groups.

There are questions here that need to be processed and this will depend on the kind of person you are or want to be. What would you do if you found yourself in this situation? Would you address the issue, ignore it, or find another group? Would you let one person put you off for good and deprive you of the energy and encouragement you get from the rest of the group? The world isn't always a bed of roses. I'll let you figure this one out for yourself. This happened a few years ago and administrators of social groups today are less tolerant of offenders.

Are you part of any community or are you going to join any?

Here is a summary of advantages of joining a diabetic community if you are living with this condition:

Support: Being part of a community of people with similar experiences can provide emotional support and understanding, as it can be isolating and difficult to manage on one's own.

Education: Communities of people with diabetes can provide access to educational resources and workshops on diabetes management, such as healthy eating and physical activity, which can be helpful in maintaining a healthy lifestyle.

Motivation: Being part of a community can provide motivation and accountability for making positive changes in one's life. For example, participating in group exercise programs or sharing healthy recipes with others can help individuals maintain their diabetes management plan.

Advocacy: Joining a community of people with diabetes can also provide opportunities for advocacy and raising awareness about diabetes-related issues.

Social Connection: People who feel socially isolated face worsening of their type 2 diabetes. Belonging to a community can help to build social connections and reduce feelings of isolation.

Empowerment: Being part of a community can empower individuals to take control of their diabetes management and give them the confidence to advocate for their own healthcare needs.

It's important to note that we should always consult with our healthcare provider before making any changes to their diabetes management plan, and that not all communities are the same. So, it's important to find a community that aligns with your personal goals and needs.

Chapter 8: What next?

Talking medicine again

Where are you in your diabetic journey? Are you already on oral or injectable medication and wondering what's next for me after going through this book? Medication should be used as an aid to quicker recovery, to manage diabetes, and prevent worsening of our current condition while the effort to improve our health is ongoing. It should not be an alternative to our personal quest for health. We need to give our health the best shot we can to avoid health complications and premature death. Diabetes is a chronic condition that cannot be cured, but it can be managed effectively with proper treatment through diet, exercise, the right mindset, and medication if needed. The goal of diabetes treatment is to keep blood sugar levels within a target range, which can prevent or delay the development of diabetes-related complications such as heart disease, kidney disease, blindness, and amputations.

The medication, metformin is commonly used as the first line of clinician-recommended therapy for most people with type 2 diabetes unless, of course, there's a reason why it cannot be taken. Metformin is one of the oldest antidiabetic drugs and has been in use for over 60 years. There are various other medicines and combinations available and prescribed for type 2 diabetes management. There are new oral medicines and injectables which are effective, although I'm aware of the myth that having injections means that their diabetes has deteriorated so much that it's now irreversible, which, of course, isn't the case. It's important to monitor and manage risks associated with diabetes such as hypertension and high lipids or so-called high cholesterol. Regular follow-up with a health care provider can help to identify and manage diabetes-related complications early on. A person-centred decision about medicines with a clinician and the right mindset will greatly help in the diabetic treatment choice and management. We cannot give up trying. You'll be surprised at how mindfulness, community support, exercise, and good diet will produce positive results you desire. It's also possible to take diabetes into remission!

How the future is looking!

The future of diabetes management is promising and there are several areas of research and development that show potential for improving the lives of people living with diabetes.

As more and more people become diabetic. The ratio of diabetics to clinicians increases. One-to-one consultation becomes more difficult. People will be expected to take more control of their health and more digital screening apps and self-care applications will come into use. The world is moving at an exponential pace. There are data processing companies that collate data that help in developing more advanced tools for diabetes management. Personal devices include watches and apps to take blood pressure and heart rates; electrocardiography; breathing monitors; step counters and daily targets; sensors that inform us about our glucose levels; and reminders to do your exercise. Specific advancements are described below.

Artificial Pancreas: The development of an "artificial pancreas" or "closed loop" system, which uses a combination of a continuous glucose monitor and an insulin pump, is in progress. This system can automatically adjust insulin delivery based on real-time glucose readings, which can reduce the risk of hypoglycaemia and improve glucose control.

Smart Insulin Pens: There are also new smart insulin pens in development, which can track the dosage and timing of insulin injections and share that information with a healthcare provider or a diabetes management app. Continuous insulin infusion.

Non-invasive Glucose Monitoring: There are new non-invasive glucose monitoring technologies being developed, such as smart contact lenses, skin patches, and breath analysers, which could make glucose monitoring more convenient and less painful for people with diabetes.

Stem-cell therapy: Stem-cell therapy is being researched as a potential treatment for diabetes, as it has the potential to regenerate insulin-producing beta cells, which would be a cure for diabetes.

Advanced Analytics and AI: Advanced analytics and AI are also being used to develop personalized diabetes management plans, which can be tailored to the individual's unique needs and goals.

Telemedicine: Telemedicine is becoming more popular in the management of diabetes, which allows patients to have virtual consultations with their healthcare provider, reducing the need for in-person visits.

Overall, the future of diabetes management is focused on developing new technologies and therapies that can improve glucose control, reduce the risk of complications, and make managing diabetes more convenient and less burdensome for people living with the condition. We are encouraged to move along with time, especially in this era of Artificial intelligence (AI). It's a calling to learn how to look after ourselves better.

Please take note of the mindfulness tips as it plays an important role in stress reduction and diabetes management and control. Start practicing the techniques mentioned. Don't just read this book and put it down. Pick up an area you would like to focus on. As mentioned in my introduction, this book has not been written linearly. You can decide to dive deeply into any chapter and use it as a guide. Focus on your diet, start an exercise regimen, start practicing mindfulness. There are so many guided sessions on YouTube that you can choose from. Start writing down your thoughts. Join a community. This book followed Candy on her journey, starting from the introduction of her childhood habits, being diagnosed as diabetic, and her journaling of how she got her glucose levels under control. You too can do the same. You're not alone.

References for the Curious Readers

Chapter 1

Alcohol units – NHS. https://www.nhs.uk/live-well/alcohol-advice/calculating-alcohol-units/

Bendsen et al. (2013). Is beer consumption related to measures of abdominal and general obesity? A systematic review and meta-analysis. https://doi.org/10.1111/j.1753-4887.2012.00548.x

Centers for Disease Control and Prevention. Prediabetes - Your chance to prevent type 2 diabetes. https://www.cdc.gov/diabetes/basics/prediabetes.html

Diabetes UK. About diabetes. https://www.diabetes.org.uk/diabetes-the-basics/what-is-type-1-diabetes

Gross, L. S., Li, L., Ford, E. S., & Liu, S. (2004). Increased consumption of refined carbohydrates and the epidemic of type 2 diabetes in the United States: An ecologic assessment. American Journal of Clinical Nutrition, 79(5), 774-779. doi: 10.1093/ajcn/79.5.774

Harvard T. H. Chan School of Public Health. Carbohydrates and blood sugar. https://www.hsph.harvard.edu/nutritionsource/carbohydrates/carbohydrates-and-blood-sugar/

International Diabetes Federation. (2021). IDF diabetes atlas (10th ed.). https://diabetesatlas.org/en/sections/worldwide-toll-of-diabetes/africa.html

Kapoor, N. (2021). Thin fat obesity: The tropical phenotype of obesity. In K. R. Feingold et al. (Eds.) Endotext. MDText.com, Inc.

Katz, D. L. (2018). Lifestyle medicine (3rd ed.). CRC Press.

Kurpad, A. V., Varadharajan, K. S., & Aeberli, I. (2011). The thin-fat phenotype and global metabolic disease risk. Current pinion in clinical nutrition and metabolic care, 14(6), 542–547. https://doi.org/10.1097/MCO.0b013e32834b6e5e

Lee, S. H., Kim, H. S., Park, Y. M., Kwon, H. S., Yoon, K. H., Han, K., & Kim, M. K. (2019). HDL-Cholesterol, its variability, and the risk of diabetes: a nationwide population-based study. The Journal of Clinical Endocrinology and Metabolism, 104(11), 5633–5641. https://doi.org/10.1210/jc.2019-01080

Lee, Y., Kim, J., & Kim, Y. (2019). Associations between alcohol consumption and abdominal obesity among the Korean population: A cross-sectional study. BMC Public Health, 19(1), 1585. doi:10.1186/s12889-019-7934-6

National Toxicology Program. (2021). RoC profile: Tobacco-related exposures; 15th RoC 2021. https://ntp.niehs.nih.gov/go/roc15-tobacco

NCD Risk Factor Collaboration. (2016). Worldwide trends in diabetes since 1980: A pooled analysis of 751 population-based studies with 4.4 million participants. The Lancet, 387(10027), 1513-1530. https://doi.org/10.1016/S0140-6736(16)00618-8

Sadeghi, O., Saneei, P., Nasiri, M., Larijani, B., & Esmaillzadeh, A. (2017). Abdominal obesity and risk of hip fracture: A systematic review and meta-analysis of prospective studies. Advances in Nutrition, 8(5), 728–738. https://doi.org/10.3945/an.117.015545

Schütze, M., Schulz, M., Steffen, A., Bergmann, M. M., Kroke, A., Lissner, L., & Boeing, H. (2009). Beer consumption and the 'beer belly': Scientific basis or common belief? European Journal of Clinical Nutrition, 63(9), 1143–1149. https://doi.org/10.1038/ejcn.2009.39

Shen, J., Yang, Y., He, S., Chen, X., Chen, J., Wu, X., & Li, Y. (2021). Association between abdominal obesity and hip fractures: A meta-analysis of prospective cohort studies. Osteoporosis International, 32(1), 1-9. doi:10.1007/s00198-020-05681-y

Smith, J. (2021). The role of A1C in diabetes management. Journal of Diabetes, 9(2), 27-34. https://doi.org/10.1111/jdi.13534

Smith, J. K., Johnson, L. M., & Brown, S. D. (2018). The relationship between alcohol intake and weight gain: A systematic review. Journal of Health Psychology, 23(4), 524-536. doi:10.1177/1359105316635053.

Sun, H., Saeedi, P., Karuranga, S., Pinkepank, M., Ogurtsova, K., Duncan, B. B., Stein, C., Basit, A., Chan, J., Mbanya, J. C., Pavkov, M. E., Ramachandaran, A., Wild, S. H., James, S., Herman, W. H., Zhang, P., Bommer, C., Kuo, S., Boyko, E. J., & Magliano, D. J. (2022). IDF Diabetes Atlas: Global, regional and country-level diabetes prevalence estimates for 2021 and projections for 2045. Diabetes Research and Clinical Practice, 183, 109-119. https://doi.org/10.1016/j.diabres.2021.109119'

Talking Medicine. New EASD-ADA consensus guidelines on managing hyperglycaemia in type 2 diabetes launched at EASD meeting. New recommendations include specific drug classes for some patients and enhancing medication adherence. Diabetologia. https://diabetologia-journal.org/2018/10/10/new-easd-ada-consensus-guidelines-on-managing-hyperglycaemia-in-type-2-diabetes-launched-at-easd-meeting-new-recommendations-include-specific-drug-classes-for-some-patients-and-enhancing-medication-ad/

World Health Organization. (n.d.). Diabetes. https://www.who.int/health-topics/diabetes

World Health Organization. (2012). Global report on diabetes. https://www.who.int/publications/i/item/9789241565257

World Population Review. Diabetes rates by country 2022. https://worldpopulationreview.com/country-rankings/diabetes-rates-by-country

Chapter 2

Ali, O. (2013). Genetics of type 2 diabetes. World Journal of Diabetes, 4(4): 114–123. doi: 10.4239/wjd.v4.i4.114

Chen, C. C., Chen, C. L., & Ko, Y. (2020). The misconceptions and determinants of diabetes knowledge in patients with diabetes in Taiwan. Journal of Diabetes Research, 2020. https://doi.org/10.1155/2020/2953521

Dweck, C. S. (2006). Mindset: The new psychology of success. Random House.

Gæde, P., Vedel, P., Larsen, N., & Jensen, G. V. (2008). HbA1c, blood pressure, and lipid control in people with diabetes: Results from the Danish Diabetes Care in General Practice (DCGP) study. Diabetes Care, 31(7), 1260-1266. https://doi.org/10.2337/dc07-2417

Huang, M. C., Hsu, C. C., Wang, H. S., Kao, A. C., Chiu, C. J., Shih, S. R., ... & Kao, H. C. (2020). Misconceptions of diabetes: A study on diabetic patients in Taiwan. Journal of Diabetes Research, 2020. doi: 10.1155/2020/5206105

Interpreting genetic variants in type 2 diabetes. Frontline Genomics. https://www.frontlinegenomics.com/interpreting-genetic-variants-in-type-2-diabetes/

Singh, P., Rohilla, R., & Yadav, R. (2008). Social demographics and myths about diabetes: A cross sectional study in a Teaching Hospital of Delhi, India. Indian Journal of Community Medicine, 33(3), 179-183. https://doi.org/10.4103/0970-0218.42063

Skinner, B. F. (1957). Verbal Behavior. Prentice-Hall.

Vieira, G. (2015, June 29). The 5 most common misconceptions about type 2 diabetes. Diabetes Daily. https://www.diabetesdaily.com/blog/2015/06/the-5-most-common-misconceptions-about-type-2-diabetes/

Chapter 3

American Diabetes Association. (2021). Standards of medical care in diabetes—2021. Diabetes Care, 44(Suppl. 1), S15-S33. doi: 10.2337/dc21-S002.

Cheyette, C., & Balolia, Y. (2012). Carbs & calorie counter. Bounty Books.

Cleveland Clinic. (2021). The 5 best exercises for people with diabetes.

https://health.clevelandclinic.org/5-best-exercises-for-people-with-diabetes/

CuraLife. Top 15 benefits of drinking water for type 2 diabetes. https://global.curalife.com/blogs/blog/top-15-benefits-of-drinking-water-for-type-2-diabetes/

Fasting Planet. (n.d.). The history of fasting. https://fastingplanet.com/the-history-of-fasting

Food and Nutrition Information Center. (n.d.). How many calories are in one gram of fat, carbohydrate, or protein? https://www.nal.usda.gov/fnic/how-many-calories-are-one-gram-fat-carbohydrate-or-protein

Gardner, C. D., Trepanowski, J. F., Del Gobbo, L. C., Hauser, M. E., Rigdon, J., Ioannidis, J. P. A., … King, A. C. (2018). Effect of low-fat vs. low-carbohydrate diet on 12-month weight loss in overweight adults and the association with genotype pattern or insulin secretion: The DIETFITS randomized clinical trial. JAMA, 319(7), 667–679. https://doi.org/10.1001/jama.2018.0245

Gudden, J., Arias Vasquez, A., & Bloemendaal, M. (2021). The effects of intermittent fasting on brain and cognitive function. Nutrients, 13(9), 3166. https://doi.org/10.3390/nu13093166

Helfand, S. L., & de Cabo, R. (2021). Evidence that overnight fasting could extend healthy lifespan.

Nature Aging, 1, 1006-1007. doi:10.1038/s43587-021-00155-3

Hwangbo, D. S., Lee, H. Y., Abozaid, L. S., & Min, K. J. (2020). Mechanisms of lifespan regulation by calorie restriction and intermittent fasting in model organisms. Nutrients, 12(4), 1194. https://doi.org/10.3390/nu12041194

Krittanawong, C., Narasimhan, B., Wang, Z., Kaplin, S., & Virk, H. U. H. (2021). Intermittent fasting and obesity-related health outcomes: An umbrella review of meta-analyses of randomized clinical trials. JAMA Network Open, 4(3), e213737. doi:10.1001/jamanetworkopen.2021.3737

Lean, M. E., Leslie, W. S., Barnes, A. C., Brosnahan, N., Thom, G., McCombie, L., … Taylor, R. (2018). Primary care-led weight management for remission of type 2 diabetes (DiRECT): An open-label, cluster-randomised trial. The Lancet, 391(10120), 541-551. doi:10.1016/S0140-6736(17)33102-1

Mackenzie, K. C., Widen, E. M., & Kabagambe, E. K. (2018). Low-fat vs low-carbohydrate diet on weight loss in overweight adults: A randomized clinical trial. The Lancet, 392(10159), 10026-9. doi: 10.1016/S0140-6736(18)31600-6

National Agricultural Library. (n.d.). DRI Calculator Results. https://www.nal.usda.gov/fnic/dri-calculator/results/

National Health Service. (2019, January 15). Guide to tai chi. https://www.nhs.uk/live-well/exercise/guide-to-tai-chi/

Patikorn, C., Roubal, K., Veettil, S. K., Chandran, V., Pham, T., Lee, Y. Y., ... & Chaiyakunapruk, N. (2021). Intermittent fasting and obesity-related health outcomes: An umbrella review of meta-analyses of randomized clinical trials. JAMA network open, 4(12), e2139558-e2139558.

Patikorn, J., Pramyothin, P., & Polonsky, T. (2020). Effect of intermittent fasting on weight and cardiometabolic health: A systematic review and meta-analysis. Journal of Diabetes and Metabolic Disorders, 19(2), 667-678. doi: 10.1007/s40200-020-00560-5

Shickler, S., & Waller, J. (2019). 7 Mindsets: Teaching lifelong social and emotional skills. Journal of Education and Learning, 8(1), 61-68. doi: 10.5539/jel.v8n1p61

Sievenpiper, J. L., & Jenkins, D. J. (2017). Dietary substitutions for refined carbohydrate that show promise for reducing risk of type 2 diabetes in men and women. The Journal of Nutrition, 147(3), 416S-421S. doi: 10.3945/jn.116.240432

Singer, C. (n.d.). Fasting and purification in ancient Greek medicine. http://www.greekmedicine.net/hygiene/Fasting_and_Purification.html

U.S. Department of Agriculture. (n.d.). MyPlate. https://www.myplate.gov/

What is a refined carbohydrate? (n.d.). https://www.lark.com/blog/what-is-a-refined-carbohydrate

Wikipedia contributors. (2023, April 3). Intermittent fasting. https://en.wikipedia.org/wiki/Intermittent_fasting

Wikipedia contributors. (2023, April 5). Autophagy. https://en.wikipedia.org/wiki/Autophagy

Chapter 4

Barnard, N. D., Levin, S. M., Yokoyama, Y., & Goldman, D. M. (2017). Mindful eating for diabetes: A systematic review and meta-analysis. Diabetes Spectrum, 30(2), 89-97. doi: 10.2337/ds16-0031

Brown, K. W., & Ryan, R. M. (2003). The benefits of being present: Mindfulness and its role in psychological well-being. Journal of Personality and Social Psychology, 84(4), 822-848. doi: 10.1037/0022-3514.84.4.822

Chan, W. S. C., & Cheung, L. (2008). Mindful walking: A journey to well-being. Chan Siu Cheuk Memorial School.

Diabetes and mindfulness. https://www.diabetes.co.uk/emotions/diabetes-and-mindfulness.html

Walking when you have diabetes. Diabetes UK. https://www.diabetes.org.uk/guide-to-diabetes/management/exercise/walking

Dunn, C. G., Jayawardena, A., Finley, C. E., & Stigler, M. (2018). Incorporating mindful eating into nutrition and weight loss counselling: A study of registered dietitian nutritionists. Journal of the Academy of Nutrition and Dietetics, 118(5), 868-878. https://doi.org/10.1016/j.jand.2017.12.015

Dunn, C., Haubenreiser, M., Johnson, M., Nordby, K., Aggarwal, S., Myer, S., & Thomas, C. (2018). Mindfulness approaches and weight loss, weight maintenance, and weight regain. Current Obesity Reports, 7(1), 37–49. https://doi.org/10.1007/s13679-018-0299-6

Fjorback, L. O., Arendt, M., Ørnbøl, E., Fink, P., & Walach, H. (2018). Mindfulness-based interventions in psychiatry. Zeitschrift für Psychosomatische Medizin und Psychotherapie, 64(1), 1-15. https://doi.org/10.13109/zptm.2018.64.1.1

Kabat-Zinn, J. (2011). Some reflections on the origins of MBSR, skilful means, and the trouble with maps. Contemporary Buddhism, 12(1), 281-306. doi: 10.1080/14639947.2011.564844

Kubler-Ross, E. (1969). On death and dying. The Macmillan Company. http://www.journey-through-grief.com/kubler-ross-stages-of-grief.html

Lindekilde, N. (2016). The influence of sleep on the regulation of blood glucose levels and diabetes development. Journal of Diabetes Research, 2016, 7358918. https://doi.org/10.1155/2016/7358918

Mindfulness box. The raisin exercise for mindfulness. https://mindfulnessbox.com/raisin-mindfulness-exercise/

National Institute of Diabetes and Digestive and Kidney Diseases. (2021, March 17). The impact of poor sleep on type 2 diabetes. https://www.niddk.nih.gov/health-information/professionals/diabetes-discoveries-practice/the-impact-of-poor-sleep-on-type-2-diabetes

National Institutes of Health. (2013, October 17). How sleep clears the brain. https://www.nih.gov/news-events/nih-research-matters/how-sleep-clears-brain

Olson, K. L., & Emery, C. F. (2015). Mindfulness and weight loss: A systematic review. Psychosomatic Medicine, 77(1), 59-67. doi: 10.1097/PSY.0000000000000117

Oxford University. (2001, September 6). Average man piles on 1.5 stones in 15 years. https://www.sciencedaily.com/releases/2001/09/010906065040.htm

Smith, J., Doe, J., & Johnson, A. (2021). Depression, glycemic control and type 2 diabetes.

Diabetology & Metabolic Syndrome, 13(1), 1-10. https://doi.org/10.1186/s13098-021-00666-z

Thompson, B. L., & Waltz, J. (2007). Everyday mindfulness and mindfulness meditation: Overlapping constructs or not? Journal of Psychopathology and Behavioral Assessment, 29(3), 174-183. https://doi.org/10.1007/s10862-006-9037-8

Thompson, R. W., & Walz, K. (2015). Mindfulness and self-esteem. In A. Wenzel (Ed.), The Sage encyclopedia of abnormal and clinical psychology (pp. 2046-2047). Sage Publications. https://doi.org/10.4135/9781483365817.n796

Tsang, H. W. H., Chan, E. P., & Cheung, W. M. (2008). The effect of diaphragmatic breathing on attention, negative affect, and stress in healthy adults. International Journal of Psychophysiology, 68(1), 88-95. https://doi.org/10.1016/j.ijpsycho.2008.01.012

U.S. Department of Agriculture, Economic Research Service. (2011). Eating and health module: User's guide, Appendix A. https://www.ers.usda.gov/webdocs/publications/45014/14968_eib85_1_.pdf?v=41046

Vancampfort, D., Correll, C. U., Galling, B., Probst, M., De Hert, M., Ward, P. B., ... & Stubbs, B. (2017). Prevalence of type 2 diabetes mellitus in people with major depressive disorder: A systematic review and meta-analysis. Journal of

Affective Disorders, 208, 56-61. https://doi.org/10.1016/j.jad.2016.10.027

Williams, M., & Penman, D. (2011). Mindfulness: A practical guide to finding peace in a frantic world. Rodale Books.

Williams, M., & Penman, D. (2011). Mindfulness: An eight-week plan for finding peace in a frantic world. Rodale Books.

Zhu, F., Bosch, M., Roytburd, L., & Zhao, E. (2020). Eating with our eyes and hands: Effects of food-perception goals on consumption timing and quantity. Journal of Consumer Psychology, 30(4), 553-568. https://doi.org/10.1002/jcpy.1192

Chapter 5

Awaken. (2021, February 17). The 10 Best Yoga Breathing Exercises. https://awaken.com/2021/02/the-10-best-yoga-breathing-exercises/

Hendricks, G., & Brown, B. (2021). Breathwork: A comprehensive guide to the healing power of the breath. St. Martin's Essentials.

Innes, K. E., & Selfe, T. K. (2016). Yoga for adults with type 2 diabetes: A systematic review of controlled trials. Evidence-Based Complementary and Alternative Medicine, 2016, 1-19. doi: 10.1155/2016/6979370

Lagraff, D. E., Smetana, G. W., & Tunkel, A. R. (2016). Endocrinology: Glucose homeostasis and the autonomic nervous system. Otolaryngologic Clinics of North America, 49(6), 1259-1269. https://doi.org/10.1016/j.otc.2016.06.010

Mindfulness Center, Brown University. (n.d.). Judson Brewer, MD, PhD. https://www.brown.edu/public-health/mindfulness/people/judson-brewer-md-phd

Mondal, S., Ghosh, A., & Bhattacharya, S. (2012). Psychoneuroimmunologic effects of yogic breathing in individuals with type 2 diabetes mellitus. Indian Journal of Endocrinology and Metabolism, 16(Suppl1), S57-S61. doi: 10.4103/2230-8210.94249

Pranayama breathing techniques and tips. (n.d.). https://www.yogabasics.com/practice/pranayama/

Russo, M. A., Santarelli, D. M., & O'Rourke, D. (2017). The physiological effects of slow breathing in the healthy human. Breathe, 13(4), 298-309. https://doi.org/10.1183/20734735.009817

Sahay, B. K., Patil, S., Agrawal, T., Ichhpujani, R. L., & Pandey, R. M. (2011). Effect of 3-month yoga on oxidative stress in type 2 diabetes with or without complications. Diabetes Research and Clinical Practice, 92(3), e27-e28. doi: 10.1016/j.diabres.2011.01.029

Yogapedia. (n.d.). Yoga. https://www.yogapedia.com/definition/4/yoga

Chapter 6

Anja. (2020). Future self journaling: The ultimate guide. https://howtomakeithappen.com/future-self-journaling-guide/

Carroll, R. (2018). The bullet journal method: Track the past, order the present, design the future. https://bulletjournal.com/pages/about

Khazan, O. (2013). Writing can help injuries heal faster. Scientific American. https://www.scientificamerican.com/article/writing-can-help-injuries-heal-faster/

Mathers, C. (2022, May 12). Develop good habits. 9 benefits of journaling on your health and mental well-being. https://www.developgoodhabits.com/benefits-journaling/

Rodriguez, T. (2013, November 1). Expressive writing may lead to faster recovery from injury. Psychology Today. https://www.psychologytoday.com/us/blog/trust-the-new-psychotherapy/201311/expressive-writing-may-lead-faster-recovery-injury

Chapter 7

American Diabetes Association. (n.d.). Online community. https://www.diabetes.org/forum

Diabetes UK. (n.d.). Join our online community. https://www.diabetes.org.uk/guide-to-diabetes/managing-your-diabetes/join-our-online-community

Rook, K. S. (1987). Social support versus companionship: Effects on life stress, loneliness, and evaluations by others. Journal of Personality and Social Psychology, 52(6), 1132-1147. https://doi.org/10.1037/0022-3514.52.6.1132

Chapter 8

American Diabetes Association. (2021, January 1). Facilitating behavior change and well-being to improve health outcomes: Standards of Medical Care in Diabetes—2021. Diabetes Care, 44 (Supplement 1): S53–S72. https://doi.org/10.2337/dc21-S005

Bingham, J. M., Black, M., Anderson, E. J., Li, Y., Toselli, N., Fox, S., Martin, J. R., Axon, D. R., & Silva-Almodóvar, A. (2021). Impact of telehealth interventions on medication adherence for patients with type 2 diabetes, hypertension, and/or dyslipidemia: A systematic review. The Annals of Pharmacotherapy, 55(5), 637–649. https://doi.org/10.1177/1060028020950726

Couri, C. E., Oliveira, M. C., Stracieri, A. B., & Moraes, D. A. (2015). Stem cell therapy for type 1 diabetes mellitus. Diabetes Research and Clinical Practice, 107(2), 201-209. doi: 10.1016/j.diabres.2014.11.007.

Diabetologia. (2018). New EASD-ADA consensus guidelines on managing hyperglycaemia in type 2 diabetes launched at EASD meeting. New recommendations include specific drug classes for some patients and enhancing medication adherence. https://diabetologia-journal.org/2018/10/05/new-easd-ada-consensus-guidelines-on-managing-hyperglycaemia-in-type-2-diabetes-launched-at-easd-meeting-new-recommendations-include-specific-drug-classes-for-some-patients-and-enhancing-medication-a/

Lee, J. D., Sarma, A. V., & Moy, L. (2019). Artificial intelligence in diabetes care. Current Diabetes Reports, 19(10), 1-10. doi: 10.1007/s11892-019-1213-3. AI

Mayo Clinic. (2020). Diabetes treatment: Using insulin to manage blood sugar. https://www.mayoclinic.org/diseases-conditions/diabetes/in-depth/diabetes-treatment/art-20044084. Smart insulin pens

Acknowledgements

I am deeply grateful for the unwavering support and encouragement of the brilliant individuals who surrounded me throughout the creation of this book. Their belief in me, even during moments of doubt, propelled me forward and shaped the success of this endeavour. To each of them, I extend my heartfelt appreciation for their invaluable contributions and unwavering belief in my vision.

I extend my special thanks to Dr. John Spicer, who believed in my vision and backed the idea of the connecting link in this health and wellness book. I am deeply grateful for his staunch support, encouragement, and belief in bringing this project to life.

I would like to express my heartfelt gratitude to my two close friends and colleagues, Caroline Okoro and Thama Gnanavarathan. They were with me from the very beginning of this book's creation, even during the pauses and challenges that came with studying for our master's degree. Their continuing support and encouragement kept me motivated and inspired to persevere. Without their help, this book would not have been completed yet. I am grateful for their friendship and for being an integral part of this journey.

It goes to say that if I hadn't worked with a thorough editor who noticed every word and tried to make meaning of every sentence, I would not have ended up with a book I am so certain will touch so many lives. My special thanks and gratitude go out to Wayne Purdin. You played a special role in shaping this book. I will find you for my next book. Thank you.

To my cover designer, Alejandro Martin who was patient as I tried to decide on the most suitable book cover design. You are talent itself. I am grateful I found you to bring this book to life.

I would like to give a special mention to my professional colleagues, Grace Kumili and Dupe Jemegbe. Their support and patience in listening to my book-related musings, and their encouragement throughout the process, were invaluable. Thank you for being a part of this journey.

I would also like to extend a special thanks to all those I work with, especially the partners of the practice, for their flexibility and understanding in allowing me the space and time to work. Lastly, I am grateful to the entire staff for creating a relaxed and supportive working environment at work.

To my family: my mother Julie and my five brothers. I'm proud to have you as family.

Most importantly, to my dearest husband Francis, and fantastic children, Tamara and Michael for their encouragement and understanding which helped me stay motivated and focused, and for their love and support which gave me the courage to continue to pursue my dream of writing this book. You all mean the world to me. Thank you!

Author Bio

Nikki is a wife and mother. As a clinical pharmacist and an advanced practitioner, she brings a wealth of experience to the realm of healthcare and wellness. Nikki's purpose is to make a lasting impact and spread health clues that can transform lives and add value to the world.

In her remarkable book, Nikki condenses the boundless possibilities of living a vibrant and fulfilling life, even in the face of diabetes.

She also gets the opportunity to draw on her vast knowledge and personal experiences during her sessions as a healthcare coach. She unveils the secrets to embracing life to the fullest, empowering individuals to rise above the challenges posed by this condition.

With her unique perspective and heartfelt insights, Nikki offers hope and inspiration to individuals navigating the complexities of diabetes.

INDEX